Managing Persistent Pain in Adolescents

Managing Persistent Pain in Adolescents
A handbook for therapists

ROSLYN ROGERS
Occupational Therapist
Royal Children's Hospital
Victoria, Australia

Foreword by
ANITA UNRUH PhD RSW OT(C) RegNS
Professor, Health and Human Performance
and Occupational Therapy
Dalhousie University
Halifax, Nova Scotia, Canada

Radcliffe Publishing
Oxford • New York

Radcliffe Publishing Ltd
18 Marcham Road
Abingdon
Oxon OX14 1AA
United Kingdom

www.radcliffe-oxford.com
Electronic catalogue and worldwide online ordering facility.

British Library Cataloguing in Publication Data

A catalogue record for this book is available from the British Library.

ISBN-13: 978 184619 012 4

Typeset by Pindar New Zealand (Egan Reid), Auckland, New Zealand
Printed and bound by TJI Digital, Padstow, Cornwall, UK

Contents

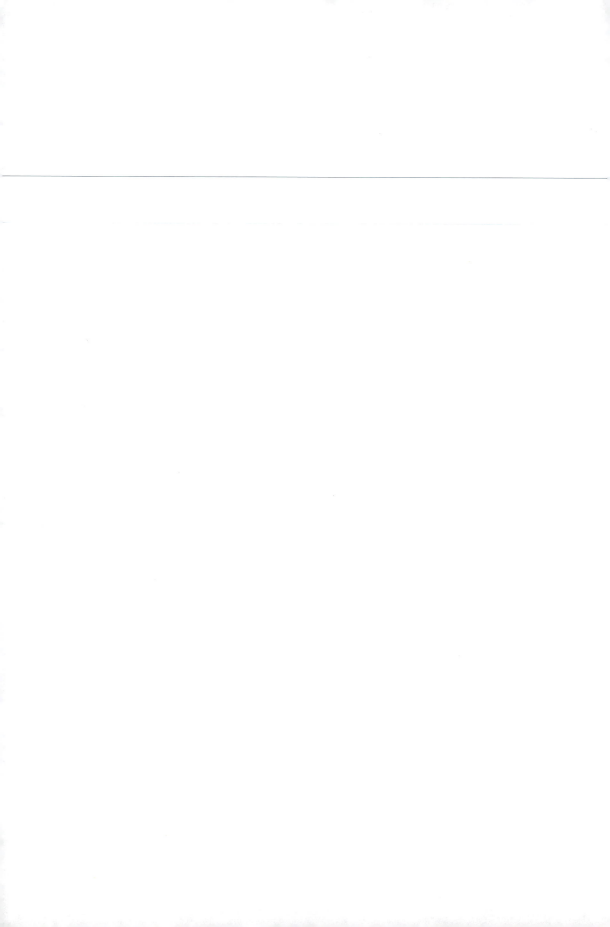

Foreword

In the past 30 years our understanding of pain in infants, children and adolescents has advanced by leaps and bounds. As a result there are many books now about pain in children, and an excellent book on pain in neonates which is now in its third edition. But there is, as yet, no book that is specifically concerned with pain in adolescents and their special needs and circumstances. More importantly, there has been no clinical book that is specifically for the therapists and practitioners who work with adolescents living with pain.

Roslyn Rogers has worked with adolescents in pain for many years in her capacity as an occupational therapist at the Royal Children's Hospital in Victoria, Australia. Rogers has always worked as a member of a multidisciplinary team using a biopsychosocial approach, and believes that a team approach will work whereas serial referrals to a single discipline are more likely to fail. This view is supported by existing pain research; implementing a biopsychosocial approach enables adolescents who have been unable to function (sometimes for years) to live a meaningful life – sometimes despite their pain, sometimes with no pain, sometimes with less pain. Rogers is convinced that therapists can assist families and adolescents to apply strategies that support optimal coping and independence.

Rogers has taken the theoretical underpinnings of cognitive behavioural therapy and contextual cognitive behavioural therapy, and applied them to the issues of adolescents as they pertain to managing and living with pain. There is a strong focus in this book on practical, applied strategies – including working with beliefs and values, mindfulness meditation, relaxation and imagery along with improving overall physical fitness and promoting routines for restorative sleep. Family relationships and the family context are always a significant issue for parents and adolescents who are struggling with significant health concerns. Rogers provides a practical discussion about interventions with families that is thoughtful, compassionate and firm in promoting the adolescent's need to take responsibility for her or his health towards independence. A significant aspect of this direction is negotiating return to school and the anxieties and uncertainties a return will hold for the adolescent and family.

Each chapter has sections that provide practical instructions and suggested ways to deal with potential obstacles. 'Yellow flags ⚷' are used to identify key psychosocial factors that may interfere for the child, family or school and some strategies for managing these factors. Clinicians will appreciate the many case examples. Many of the cases are success stories but others illustrate the complexity of situations that do not resolve or improve easily, if at all, and some of the issues that can limit progress.

This book is a wonderful clinical book for those who are interested in understanding more about the practical application of contextual cognitive behavioural therapy for the management of pain in adolescents.

Anita Unruh
Professor, Health and Human Performance and Occupational Therapy
Dalhousie University
Halifax, Nova Scotia, Canada
January 2008

Preface

For the last eight years I have been treating adolescents with persistent pain who have been referred to a multidisciplinary outpatient pain management clinic attached to a large paediatric hospital. The multidisciplinary team in the clinic consists of an occupational therapist, a physiotherapist, a psychologist, an anaesthetist and a consultant psychiatrist and follows a consistent programme based on cognitive behaviour therapy. The pain management outpatient clinic is open to all children up to 18 years of age. Most of our population are adolescents with a mean age of 14 years. For this reason this book is based on an adolescent population.

The idea for this book has grown in my mind for some years. The impetus grew whenever I had students or a health practitioner just starting practice, or phone calls from solo practitioners, particularly in rural areas, struggling to understand what to *do* with an adolescent whose pain and distress was greater than the original injury: 'they 'ought' to be better', 'it's a mystery', 'it's all psychological', 'we've tried this, we've tried that, nothing works' being recurring themes. The impetus also grew whenever our team failed in our attempts to find a therapist or therapists able to treat persistent pain not as unimodal but as a complex biopsychosocial problem. We have always needed a support system of therapists in the community to whom our patients could be referred following completion of our programme.

Finally, as I worked in a teaching hospital with access to training and libraries, I dreamt of providing a bridge between the academic arm of research in the pain-management specialty and the clinical application of these ideas. Most therapists in the community do not have either time or access to conferences, journals and books. Additionally, knowledge in chronic pain management is drawn from a very wide field. For this reason, I have made an attempt to support suggestions for clinical practice with evidence from a wide field. Sometimes, however, there is no clear evidence for what is common clinical practice. This does not mean that a practice is inadvisable: it may reflect the insufficiency of evidence or the limitations of scientific investigation. Therefore, some suggestions in this book are based on clinical experience while others are based on evidence presented in the research literature, and this is indicated in the text. While the book does not critically appraise the literature, there are some meta-analyses and reviews contained in the references.

Writing this book has been a natural outcome of my accumulated experiences. This experience has been gained not just as part of a multidisciplinary team in an outpatient clinic for adolescents with persistent pain, but also as a yoga teacher and an occupational therapist in both physical and psychiatric settings – including return-to-work rehabilitation programmes for adults with chronic pain. In the past, I have been a classroom teacher and have taught yoga and creative dance to adults and children.

An equally significant motivation for writing this book is a stubborn belief that practitioners of all 'disciplines' that are likely to be called upon to treat an adolescent with persistent pain need, to some extent, to step outside their discipline and acquire interdisciplinary skills. For instance, what is required are physiotherapists with the ability to work psychologically; psychologists who can incorporate physical goals, and occupational therapists who work with family issues that impact on pain.

The descriptor *persistent* rather than *chronic* is used to describe longstanding pain, for a number of reasons. The permanent changes in the pain system of adults with longstanding pain that legitimise the concept of chronic pain as a disease state have not been shown in children and adolescents. 'Persistent' pain implies recognition of the recurring nature of the past pain without predicting the nature of the pain in the future, thereby offering the prospect of a more positive future.

Prior to referral to the clinic, our patients have frequently seen a variety of medical specialists including rheumatologists; orthopaedic surgeons; urologists; gynaecologists; gastroenterologists; neurologists; ear, nose and throat specialists, and ophthalmologists, to name but a few. They may also have seen alternative specialists including osteopaths; naturopaths; chiropractors; kinaesiologists; faith healers; acupuncturists, or Chinese herbalists. Finally, they are likely to have consulted their general practitioner who may have referred them to their local physiotherapist, counsellor, psychologist or occupational therapist.

It is also apparent that many of the adolescents we see have had serial referrals from one discipline to another, each assessing and treating one particular aspect of the whole picture – this is rather like the well-known story of a group of individuals each examining parts of an elephant without anyone describing the whole animal. The issues associated with adolescents with persistent pain are complex, interwoven problems that are psychological, social and biological and that need to be addressed as a whole.

This book will provide some practical suggestions to all those therapists involved in the treatment of adolescents with persistent pain.

Roslyn Rogers
January 2008

Acknowledgements

I would like to acknowledge the assistance of those people who have been kind enough to read for me chapters within their specialty areas of psychology and physiotherapy: the team at Bath Pain Management Program and in particular the team members who have worked with me over the years at The Royal Children's Hospital Pain Management Clinic: Mark Bradford, Brendon Egan, Sophia Franks, Dr George Chalkiadis, Andrea Campbell, Anna Young and Megan Turville. I would also like to thank my husband for his constant support and encouragement.

This book is dedicated to the adolescents and their families who present to the clinic and who face their difficulties with commitment and courage.

They continue to inspire and teach me.

Using this book

Who can use it?

This book is written for therapists or clinical practitioners who are not necessarily specialised in the management of persistent pain but who find themselves treating an adolescent with persistent or chronic pain. Any therapist that is caring for such an adolescent will find this book useful. Therapists such as occupational therapists, psychologists and physiotherapists will find that it extends aspects of their existing training beyond the bounds of their discipline. Additionally, I hope other clinical practitioners – including nurses, social workers, osteopaths, acupuncturists and counsellors – will use this book to extend their understanding of what may be helpful for an adolescent in their care who suffers from persistent pain. Physicians who are interested in knowing about appropriate referrals for therapy will also find it useful.

This book is for therapists who wish to help adolescents find or regain a fulfilling life, in which they are not a victim to pain and where pain is not in charge of their lives. It is not about magic cures for pain.

The theoretical model

The theoretical model for the book is cognitive behavioural therapy (CBT) with reference to contextual cognitive behavioural therapy (CCBT). A recent description and justification for its application in adolescents with persistent pain is to be found in the Introduction. In brief, CBT appear to have the greatest body of evidence, however limited in scope, to support its use in the management of persistent pain in adolescents with headaches.[1,2] Although there are other theoretical models for treatment, it is not within the scope of this book to address these.

How to use this book

The book is divided into three sections. Each section has chapters that address separate topics likely to arise in the course of a therapist's work. Therapists may deal with more than one aspect simultaneously when dealing with an adolescent and his or her family. The first chapter discusses the engagement process for the adolescent and family. The therapist needs to be aware that family issues outlined in the first section of Chapter 1 may need to be dealt with later after some trust has been established. The first section (Chapters 1–4) shows how the therapist can use information about pain, its causes and diagnosis, to assist the family and the adolescent. This section includes chapters which identify complicating factors in the adolescent's environment that contribute to the complex picture of the adolescent with persistent pain. The second section (Chapters 5–8) deals with managing pain and the factors that influence motivation and coping. The third section (Chapters 9–10) addresses the practical issues of physically re-engaging in life activities.

Questionnaire

If the therapist has a specific adolescent in mind, it will be useful to complete the questionnaire at the end of this section. The questionnaire will help to target areas of treatment immediately useful to their patient.

Case studies

Case studies are used throughout the book to illustrate points made in the chapters. Some of these demonstrate the 'yellow flag' (see below) that may arise in treating an adolescent and their family. These cases are chosen to demonstrate the complexity and reality of clinical practice. The reality of clinical practice is that outcomes are dependent on the therapist, the treating team, the adolescent, and the family – a complex mix of factors that includes personalities, personal skills and motives, as well as medical and environmental factors. Case studies depict the complexities of the process of pain management and highlight possible negative outcomes from 'yellow flags' (see below). Case studies are cross-referenced if they are referred to in more than one chapter.

'Yellow flags' and 'red flags'

As pain is multifactorial, there are many areas that can thwart a physical-based rehabilitation. 'Yellow flag' or 'red flag' will alert the practitioner to these barriers.[3] 'Yellow flags' identify psychosocial factors that may influence recovery, while 'red flags' indicate a serious underlying medical condition requiring urgent attention. Examples of physical signs likely to affect recovery may be a sustained increase in swelling, or temperature changes of a joint or limb. These are likely to require a consultation with the treating medical practitioner.

This handbook is not designed to diagnose or treat medical conditions and therefore does not cover the full range of signs to which a therapist may need to be alert, as these may include underlying neurological pathology, tumours, infections, rheumatological or orthopaedic conditions. For this reason, 'red flags' as such are not identified in the book. However the treating therapist needs to be alert to physical changes and to maintain close communication with an overseeing doctor. It is essential to have appropriate medical information that indicates medical status and that indicates whether all investigations have been completed. Even with appropriate medical information, new pathology may be discovered. Doubts or new developments need to be discussed with the overseeing doctor as they occur in treatment.

As pain has many factors which simultaneously impact on the adolescent and their family, it is often useful to address many areas at the same time. A team with several practitioners taking different roles who maintain close communication works most effectively.[4] The success of one aspect of treatment may depend on another aspect being addressed first. This is discussed within particular chapters.

Definitions

The International Association for the Study of Pain (IASP) Task Force on taxonomy has produced clear definitions and classifications of chronic pain. It is therefore unnecessary to reproduce these in this handbook, and the reader is referred to the IASP's excellent definitions and classifications which promote the standardisation of taxonomy.[5]

A questionnaire for therapists

This questionnaire alerts the therapist to possible problem areas. If several of these answers are in the affirmative, a full biopsychosocial assessment is required.

	YES/NO	CHAPTER(S)
Has your patient had pain for longer than three months?		1 and 2
Have single treatment modalities been unsuccessful, e.g. physiotherapy, counselling?		Introduction
Does the pain seem out of proportion to the original diagnosis?		1, 6 and 8
Is the underlying cause of the pain understood?		1 and 2
Has the pain caused significant disruption to the young person's or their family's life?		3
Do family members need to modify what they do to accommodate the needs of the young person? (For example, massage him/her, stay at home, leave events early.)		1 and 3
Have the adolescent's fitness levels reduced since the onset of pain?		5 and 9
Does the adolescent lie down or sleep during the day?		4, 5 and 9
Does the young person frequently express his/her pain?		3, 7 and 8
Does the adolescent concentrate on, or seem worried about his/her body sensations?		7
Does the young person talk about his/her pain in colourful or extreme terms or images?		8
Is there sleep disturbance?		4
Have the adolescent's social contacts or activities changed because of pain?		5
Is school attendance a problem?		10
Have parents or grandparents needed to stay at home to be with the adolescent?		3

A more comprehensive aid to assessing outcomes is the Bath Adolescent Pain Questionnaire (BAPQ), which assesses many of the areas addressed throughout this handbook, i.e. physical functioning, social functioning, depression, general anxiety, pain-specific anxiety, family functioning, and development in adolescents.[6]

References

1 Eccleston C, Morley S, Williams A, *et al*. Systematic review of randomised controlled trials of psychological therapy for chronic pain in children and adolescents, with a subset meta-analysis of pain relief. *Pain.* 2002; **99**: 157–65.

2 Eccleston C, Merlijn VPBM, Hunfeld JAM. Translating evidence for psychological interventions to manage recurrent pain and chronic pain in children and adolescents: three trials. In: Dostrovsky JO, Carr DB, Koltzenburg M, editors. Proceedings of the 10th World Congress on Pain. *Progress in Pain Research and Management*; 2003; **24**: 853–62.

3 Australian Acute Musculoskeletal Pain Guidelines Group. *Evidence-based Management of Acute Musculoskeletal Pain: a guide for clinicians.* Bowen Hills, Queensland, Australia: Australian Academic Press; 2004.

4 Flor H, Fydrich R, Turk D. Efficacy of multidisciplinary pain treatment centers: a meta-analytic review. *Pain.* 1992; **49**: 221–30.

5 http://www.iasp-pain.org//AM/Template.cfm?Section=Home

6 Eccleston C, Jordan A, McCracken L. The Bath Adolescent Pain Questionnaire (BAPQ): development and preliminary psychometric evaluation of an instrument to assess the impact of chronic pain on adolescents. *Pain.* 2005; **118**(1–2): 163–270.

Note

The handouts in the Appendix are also available to download and print off at www.radcliffe-oxford.com/adolescentpain.

Introduction

For some, pain is not a passing experience that disappears with the healing of damaged tissue or when a danger has passed. Persistent pain continues to have a constant and debilitating effect on the lives of those who have it and on those around them.

In parents' words . . .
'It's torture, you just wish that, you know, you could take it away from them and you can't, and its not just frustration, it's worse than frustration I think. It's like being tortured.'

'Its amazing how exhausting it is . . . mentally, emotionally and physically, I would never have believed it . . . We're through that phase now . . . but I remember how incredibly tired I got. If I sat down, I would go to sleep.'

'And do you know the way you're often waiting for a bone scan or an X-ray and nobody had believed you . . . God forgive me, I prayed. I hoped that something would be on it.'

'I think that for me it's what the future holds . . . I don't dwell on it . . . but I think it's . . . it's you know, what's next?'[1]

In adolescents' words . . .
'It's frustrating not to be able to do normal things.'

'I just want it to go away.'

'It's the most awful thing that has happened to me.'

Those who experience persistent pain, or who are closely associated with a young person living with persistent pain, know it can affect nearly every aspect of their life: mood; the ability to sleep; concentration, and hence academic performance. It affects friendships, social events and family relationships – not to mention the daily activities so much taken for granted in normal childhood:

play, favourite sports, hobbies, even independent self-care. For each family and adolescent, the story will be different in detail but the principle is the same. Pain can evoke a multiplicity of feelings in adults (teachers; parents; older siblings) responsible for those children: anger, fear, indignation, guilt, blame, sadness, even hopelessness. A large amount of adults' time may be spent attempting to prevent and relieve the pain. When this apparently fails, it is often difficult to get a perspective that is beyond these often overpowering feelings. Pain has become the 'boss' of their lives. The young person is blamed, parents are blamed, therapists and doctors are blamed. Parents, teachers and carers need help in understanding how pain works and knowing what to do to help (*see* Chapters 6 and 8).

There are a number of studies that highlight the incidence and dysfunction in adolescents with chronic or recurrent pain.[2,3]

1   The incidence of chronic or recurrent pain in children and adolescents in the population is 15%, with girls reporting more pain than boys. The incidence in the paediatric population equals the incidence in the adult population.
2   The incidence of reported chronic pain peaks at age 14 years. (This handbook is targeted to this age group.)
3   During the time spent in a 'diagnostic vacuum', the child 'often receives little appropriate pain management' (pain management strategies are addressed in Chapters 6, 7, and 8, while Chapter 2 deals with the 'diagnostic vacuum').
4   They develop 'chronic physical disability, anxiety, sleep disturbance, school absence, and social withdrawal'. (*See* Chapters 4, 8, 9 and 10.)
5   'Parents report severe parenting stress and dysfunctional family roles.' (*See* Chapter 3.)
6   Families interpret inaccurate diagnoses such as 'functional' or 'psycho-somatic' as blaming them for their child's pain. (*See* Chapters 1 and 2.)
7   'A child with chronic pain who does not respond to simple first-line treatment requires the input of an interdisciplinary team of therapists trained in the management of pain.' (*See* all chapters.)
8   'More action is necessary . . . more paediatric centres are needed, to develop chronic pain programmes.'[4]

Adolescence

Adolescence is that significant stage of transition between the dependence of childhood and the independence expected in adulthood. While adolescence is defined loosely in this book, as the period in a person's life between 11 and 20 years of age, actual maturation into adulthood is a complex interaction of physical, social and emotional processes that is not easily defined by an exact age limit. Many 'adults' may continue to exhibit behaviour that is socially and emotionally 'immature' after the physical maturity of adulthood has been reached. Adolescence is a time when many expectations are placed upon the young person, and when they themselves are envisaging their future, for better or for worse. They may place undue expectations on themselves, as may their parents or social group. Biologically as well as socially and emotionally, they are in an intense state of readiness for, and actual change. They are at a stage when they are learning new skills, testing their efficacy in life generally and learning their personal strengths and weaknesses. They are measuring their performance against that of their peers and facing the process of defining themselves and their values as an individual. In particular, they are deciding in what ways they want to be different from or the same as their adult role models, their parents.

There are many points of transition in the adolescent stage: transition from one school to another; from school to higher education; from pre-pubescent to active sexuality; from primarily parent influence to peer influence. Transitions have a number of characteristics.[5]

- An eager anticipation of the future.
- A sense of regret for the stage that has been lost.
- A feeling of anxiety in relation to the future.
- A major psychological readjustment.
- A degree of ambiguity of status during the transition.

Adolescence is described as the second phase of individuation. The first stage is completed with the separation phase of infancy and the attainment of self and object constancy – the 'I' and 'not I' by the age of four years.[6] In adolescent development, the individuation process may be defined as an equilibrating process between connectedness and individuality within the family. The adolescent is negotiating a path within existing family relationships, by seeking to make individual choices that may not necessarily be in agreement (with those of parents in particular), and which may be a departure from established family rules – thereby establishing their individuality while maintaining their relationships.

Parents

Parents of an individuating adolescent are also in a state of change, as they negotiate this path. They too, are envisaging the end of their child's childhood, and their future in this picture. In this context a first, last or only child is likely to have greater significance for a parent. They may have complex emotions that are not articulated even to themselves; emotions such as regret, sadness or fear. Issues of separation anxieties that existed during an earlier transition time of individuation, for example at first-time kindergarten or school attendance, are likely to resurface in the face of their child's increasing independence. They may worry that their child will not cope without them. Each child's place in the family places different experiences on parent and child. The experience of a first child's adolescence is likely to be different from the experience of the last child's. For example, the first-time parent may experience a loss of control as their child challenges their authority and tests their boundaries of behaviour. Parents may discover a need for boundaries they have been unable to establish in earlier years. New parenting skills of negotiation are required and a different relationship to their child is required of them. A parent of the last child may fear that their life without a dependent child will be meaningless or lonely. A spectrum of these scenarios may occur in the general population with varying degrees of successful transition into adulthood. This period can be stressful in itself for a parent. Having an adolescent with persistent pain is an additional stress that compounds these pre-existing issues. Although the gaining of independence is a process that does not start at the age of 11 years, parents of a younger, more dependent child can feel more secure in their authority as parents, before their authority is questioned in the later adolescent stage.

Considerable evidence exists supporting the stress experienced by parents of adolescents who experience persistent or chronic pain.[7] There are a number of interesting factors identified. Parents report a belief that their children complain of pain in order to avoid non-preferred activity. Equally, over-attentiveness reinforces pain complaint and disability. Adolescents report receiving less attention for their pain behaviour from peers than from parents. Adolescents with persistent pain are exposed to a higher number of adults with pain behaviour. The parental skills required for this age group differ from those needed in the case of the younger child. The parental role is different from the role of partners of adults with chronic pain. What this means for the therapist is that each family requires individual assessment and individual guidance regarding appropriate responses for pain in their child.

Treatment
The role of the therapist
Pain in a patient or client can trigger many feelings in the therapist. There may be annoyance that this patient is not coping, whereas others with the same condition have been able to. Another feeling may be a desire to be the hero or advocate to the suffering child. Obviously, neither of these feelings is helpful: the first is unhelpful because blaming does not assist in finding a solution and guiding therapy; the second is unhelpful because fundamental to ongoing success of pain management is that the adolescent perceives that the success of therapy has been dependent on their independent effort. It is, after all, in the application of strategies *outside* of the therapy sessions that really counts.

Empowering the adolescent to take effective action is fundamental to the role of the therapist. Of necessity this involves teaching strategies so that the adolescent will not only understand what increases pain (such as pacing (*see* Chapter 9)), but also know how to move towards a fulfilling life (*see* Chapter 5) despite ongoing pain or pain flare-ups (*see* Chapters 6 and 8).

Whatever the nature of the adolescent's pain, a detailed understanding of the individual's pain is necessary at the outset. (*See* 'Assessment' in Chapter 1.) Pain can be constant, as in a chronic daily tension headache, or it can flare up for minutes, hours or days. Recognising patterns of pain can be of assistance in identifying triggers such as classroom or playground difficulties, anxieties, or school refusal (*see* Chapter 10). For some however, there is no discernable pattern in pain flare-up. Accepting the unpredictability of the flare-ups without being stalemated by 'why' may be part of managing helpful/unhelpful thoughts (*see* Chapters 2 and 8).

Teamwork

A multidisciplinary team consisting of a pain specialist anaesthetist, a physio-therapist, an occupational therapist, a psychologist and a consultant psychiatrist will cover the necessary areas in the pain-management specialty area. Close teamwork involving shared assessment, discussion, case formulation and implementation of the treatment plan ensures consistency of treatment. Of necessity there is an overlap of roles. For example, the physiotherapist may work with either the psychologist or the occupational therapist in mindfulness techniques during their session. All therapists may share the goal setting process. The education session may be jointly presented and may be referred to by all treating clinicians. The use of shared language and metaphors by all team members provides consistency and reinforcement for the adolescent and family.

However, in the absence of the ideal team, it may still be possible to share some of the suggestions put forward in this book with therapists or clinicians (and these may include doctors) operating separately.

A biopsychosocial model of pain

There are many ways of approaching the problem of chronic pain and the distress and disability associated with it. The notion of pain as bio-medical model is that pain is either 'physical', with pain consistent with the pathology, the degree of damage or disease, or, if the pain is inconsistent with underlying pathology then the pain is deemed to be 'psychological' pain. This bio-medical model frequently leads to the person with unexplained persistent pain feeling that they are not believed or that they are sent to the psychologist as a last resort due to failure of traditional medical methods. They may also feel that the medical practitioners consider their pain as not real, felt pain; the pain may have been described as psychosomatic or 'in the head'. This bio-medical model has been discounted on many fronts including in terms of current information from neurobiology and social research.

Information from neurobiology now supports the biopsychosocial model of chronic pain, confirming the interrelationship of biology (including the influence of genetic and developmental factors on a 'plastic' nervous system) with the psychological and social development of the individual (*see* Chapter 1).

The population of adolescents with persistent pain has factors that determine or maintain chronic pain. There are higher levels of negative effect and fear of failure; greater use of emotion-focused avoidance; coping strategies, and less strong perceptions that they are socially accepted.[8]

The cognitive-behavioural perspective

There is evidence for cognitive behavioural therapy (CBT) as a treatment for individuals with chronic or persistent pain.[9,10] The cognitive-behavioural perspective on chronic pain is that individuals actively seek to make sense of their experience by appraising their condition. For this reason, education on the condition (persistent pain) is an initial part of a CBT programme as presented in Chapters 1 and 2.[11] Cognitive behavioural therapy incorporates concepts from the learning theories articulated by early behaviouralists (Pavlov, Watson, Skinner, Wolpe, Bandura and Cautela). As early as 1976, Wilbert Fordyce used operant behavioural methods (first described by Skinner) with adult chronic pain patients targeting excessive pain behaviour and the absence of wellness behaviour. He identified the role that exposure to systematic contingencies of reinforcement in the environment played in the behaviour.

Concepts of the early behaviouralist that have become part of the lexicon of therapists and an educated public are: *conditioned responses, reinforcement, extinguishment, desensitisation*. Additionally, concepts arising from social learning theory include *modelling* as learning, and learning by *imagining* and *rehearsing*. While it is beyond the scope of this book to elaborate on these theories, it is appropriate to understand these concepts as they are central to a CBT pain management programme. For instance, in Chapter 3 on 'Pain and the family', there is a discussion about learned pain behaviour that may arise from *modelling* within a family where other members also experience pain. Pain behaviour may be *positively reinforced* by rewards such as massages, attention of a loved one, or staying home from school. In Chapter 5, 'Making changes', strategies are mentioned that may include uses of *imagining* change in the goal-setting process and *rehearsing* in managing peer relations at school by role playing with the therapist.

Other theorists have developed important concepts relevant to the management of pain, namely self-efficacy (Bandura) and the role of appraisals in coping (Folkman and Lazarus).[12,13]

Cognitive behavioural therapy (CBT) and the more recent development of contextual cognitive behavioural therapy (CCBT) are the most commonly researched treatments in the field of pain management. CCBT identifies key areas of difference from CBT while acknowledging a common heritage and shared techniques. The following is a brief description of that common heritage and new developments. Fuller reading in this area is recommended.[14,15]

Cognitive behavioural therapy (CBT)

Traditionally, CBT accepts the phenomenological nature of an individual's experience and therefore the content of their cognitions, sometimes called automatic thoughts or self-talk. CBT focuses on providing information on the condition and on the relationship between thoughts, body responses and behaviour (e.g. fearful thoughts that produce a racing heart or shakiness or increased pain that lead to withdrawal from activity). Patients are then taught mechanisms to relieve symptoms in the body by techniques such as relaxation or breathing. Treatment includes assessment of the 'dysfunctional' automatic thoughts and self-statements and a focus on reframing or restructuring these, i.e. by changing the content, frequency or form of thoughts and beliefs. This process challenges the logic, likelihood or helpfulness of the thoughts. CBT works with ways to challenge or change thoughts that are unhelpful. This has been described as reappraisal or reconceptualising the problem. Behavioural experiments such as graduated exposure may also occur in a CBT.

Contextual cognitive behavioural therapy

Contextual cognitive behavioural therapy (CCBT) has been described as one of the 'third wave' behavioural therapies along with **dialectical behaviour therapy, mindfulness-based therapy** and **acceptance commitment therapy**. As therapies in the field of pain management, CBT and CCBT are the most commonly researched treatments.

The goal of CCBT therapy is for the patient/client to live a life of fulfilment and vitality whatever sensations are present at the time. In this process, symptoms may lessen but the goal is not to diminish 'symptoms' such as pain or other unpleasant internal events such as thoughts, feelings or sensations.

CCBT arises from the empirically based relational frame theory (RFT), a theory on the acquisition and function of language in humans. Language (which includes gesture and imagery as well as cognitions) was developed to anticipate and solve *problems* around food, water, shelter, sex and, above all, survival. People use language to make maps and models of the world, predict and plan for the future and share knowledge. This process allows us to learn from the past, imagine, create, communicate, and learn from people who are no longer alive. The negative side of language produces libel, slander, ignorance, criticism and condemnation; dwells on and re-lives painful events in memories, and creates ineffective rules for ourselves.

Relational frame theory (RFT) describes ways in which networks of historically conditioned verbal relations are acquired, the negative content of which is difficult to alter because the relational networks work by addition not by subtraction. They are therefore not open to content-focused change (i.e. the traditional focus of change described previously in CBT). This notion of addition is the basis of *acceptance* of recurring unpleasant thoughts and sensations – a key notion underpinning the third wave therapies.

Therapy

Therapy focuses on *acceptance* of negative thoughts, emotions and sensations, including pain. These are collectively known as 'unwanted private events'. These unwanted private events are beyond personal control, being unresponsive to verbal controls such as 'I must not think about pain'. CCBT is interested in the *function* of clinically problematic behaviours, i.e. what the thought, emotion impulse behaviour is in the service of, rather than its form; how frequently it occurs, or whether it is logical.

For some adolescents who experience chronic or persistent pain, the attempt to control or avoid these unwanted private events (sensations, thoughts, images) causes avoidance behaviours that are the source of their dysfunction, i.e. withdrawal from social or physical activities.

Therapy consists of working with the person to recognise their unwanted private events (*see* Chapter 7 on mindfulness training) with acceptance rather than avoidance of these unwanted internal events. Mindfulness training teaches the adolescent to see their negative internal events as transient, to name them as memories, old stories, etc.; to 'defuse' from them and lessen their power over the adolescent's actions by simply observing them as they occur in the moment. In this process, the adolescent establishes a sense of self that is less enmeshed and is separate from their negative influence. This then allows different choices to be made that are not avoidant. Behavioural experiments such as graduated exposure to events previously avoided may also occur in mindfulness training.

Identifying *values* that the adolescent wants their actions to reflect, assists them to make different choices for their actions. For instance, questions to ask may be: 'How would you like friends and family to see you; what sort of person do you want to **be**?' 'Does this action fit in with this?' These questions are different from the question, 'What do you want to **do**?' (*see* Chapter 5).

Common ground

Common ground between CCBT and CBT is that the therapist becomes a partner in the therapy process rather than the person who hold the answers which they will give out (usually in a didactic form) to the person presenting for treatment. In CBT and CCBT discoveries and learning are achieved by shared enquiry.

CCBT proposes a treatment programme that focuses on recognition and redefinition of the 'agenda' (the agenda is usually avoidance of unwanted private events), awareness and acceptance of unpleasant private events, and assistance in making behavioural choices that are not driven by these internal events.

Assistance in making behavioural choice is in the form of working with the patient to identify values, recognising the existence of an 'observer self' through mindfulness activities, giving assistance in the separation or 'defusion' with private events. The patients are then more able to be 'present in the moment' (context) and to choose actions that are committed in the direction of their values. Repeating this process of committed actions builds an expanding base of values-based actions.

CCBT makes use of traditional techniques such as graduated exposure, sensate focus, etc. but for different ends – i.e. not for the diminution of negative private events but for 'willingness' to have them while taking values-based action.

Eight basic strategies identified
- Confronting the agenda (creative hopelessness, what it has cost you).
- Control is the problem. (What has been tried? Has it worked?)
- Cognitive defusion (thoughts as bits of language passing through, as opposed to thoughts as reality).
- Acceptance (willingness is an alternative to control).
- Contacting the present moment (thoughts are like a radio messages that one can observe).
- Self as context (a sense of self as the context in which negative private events occur, like the weather changes that occur in the 'context' of the sky).
- Valuing as a choice (knowing what sort of person you want to be and making behavioural choices that do what complies with identified values).
- Commitment and action. (Commitment to build larger patterns of values-based action. It is not a promise or prediction of a particular outcome, but a commitment.)

What is achievable from treatment

Initially the agenda of the adolescent and family may be to get rid of or control the pain. Addressing this agenda is part of the early stage of treatment. It is important that the therapist and adolescent have an understanding of what to expect as an outcome from treatment. The adolescent and family have usually tried in many ways to do this before presenting for treatment and have not succeeded. It is this agenda that has most often led to many avoidant activities (resting, staying at home, etc.) that have resulted in a diminished and restricted lifestyle for the young person and the family.

The aim of treatment is to restore a fulfilling lifestyle by allowing the adolescent to accept whatever unpleasant and uncontrollable experiences life offers (including pain) and to learn to live in accordance with their personal values by taking action accordingly. This may mean proceeding with chosen activity despite pain, worry, etc. What follows is likely to be a fulfilling life which may or may not include levels of pain or other negative internal physical or emotional experiences. Of course, using the strategies suggested throughout this book may reduce pain. A commonly expressed outcome is, 'Yes, I do still have some pain but it doesn't bother me like it used to.'

This book shows strategies for presenting this discussion and strategies for learning acceptance and commitment in therapy and life outside therapy.

Of course, some adolescents and families are not ready for this treatment and will continue to seek treatment or personal actions that will attempt to control pain. Some case studies exemplify this (*see* Chapter 3 'Case study: James').

References

1 Jordan AL, Eccleston C, Osborn M. Being a parent of the adolescent with complex chronic pain: an interpretative phenomenological analysis. *Eur J Pain.* 2007; **11**: 49–56.
2 Perquin CW, Hazebroek-Kampschreur AAJM, Hunfield JAM, *et al.* Pain in children and adolescents: a common experience. *Pain.* 2000; **87**: 51–8.
3 Merlijn VPBM, Munfeld JAM, van der Wouden JC, *et al.* Psychosocial factors associated with chronic pain in adolescents. *Pain.* 2003; **101**(1–2): 33–43.
4 Eccleston C. Managing chronic pain in children and adolescents. *BMJ.* 2003; **326**: 1408–9, doi: 10.1136/bmj.326.7404.1408.
5 Coleman JC, Hendry LB. *The Nature of Adolescence,* 3rd ed. London, New York: Routledge; 1999.
6 Blos P. *The Adolescent Passage,* 2nd ed. New York: NY International Universities Press; 1979.
7 Hunfeld JAM, Perquin CW, Hasebroek-Kampschreur AAJM, *et al.* Physically unexplained chronic pain and its impact on children and their families: their mother's perception. *Psychol Psychother Theory Res Pract.* 2002; **75**: 251–60.
8 Merlijn VPBM, Hunfield JAM, van der Wouden JC, *et al.* Psychosocial factors associated with chronic pain in adolescents. *Pain.* 2002; **101**: 33–43.
9 Eccleston C, Malleson PN, Clinch J, *et al.* Chronic pain in adolescents: evaluation of a programme of interdisciplinary cognitive behaviour therapy. *Arch Dis Child.* 2003; **88**(10): 881–5.
10 Jensen MP, Nielson WR, Romano JM, *et al.* Patient beliefs predict patient functioning: further support for a cognitive-behavioural model of chronic pain. *Pain.* 1999; **81**: 95–104.
11 Moseley G, Nicholas MK, Hodges PW. A randomized controlled trial of intensive neuro-physiology education in chronic low back pain. *Clinical J Pain.* 2004; **20**(5): 324–30.
12 Bandura A. *Social Foundations of Thought and Action: a social cognitive theory.* Englewood Cliffs, NJ: Prentice-Hall; c. 1986.
13 Lazarus RS, Folkman S. *Stress Appraisal and Coping.* New York: Springer; 1984.
14 McCracken LM. *Contextual Cognitive-Behavioural Therapy for Chronic Pain.* Seattle: IASP Press; 2005.
15 Hayes S, Strosahl K, editors. *A Practical Guide to Acceptance and Commitment Therapy.* New York: Springer; 2004.

CHAPTER 1

The how and why of pain

EDUCATING ABOUT PAIN AND WHAT INFLUENCES IT

CHAPTER SUMMARY

This chapter presents a biopsychosocial assessment as the basis for case formulation. It includes suggestions for preparing the family and adolescent, and a suggested format for the content of the assessment with brief discussion on some details. A grid summarises biopsychosocial factors likely to influence pain. Evidence for the value of pain physiology education is presented with suggestions for preparing the family and adolescent. An outline of the likely content of such a session is given. This is in dialogue form with questions and hypothetical answers to encourage engagement of participants in discussion. A brief summary for the family of what to expect from other sessions is described. Finally, the chapter includes a case study.

Background

Before any engagement in a treatment programme, it is necessary to fully assess all aspects of the adolescent, their family, the pain and the impact of the pain on all concerned. This biopsychosocial assessment is the basis of a case formulation and will inform treatment direction.

A biopsychosocial assessment involves the gathering of information that assists the therapist to understand the biological basis for the pain as well as psychological and social influences. Biological factors may include medical events or injuries prior to the presenting condition, perhaps in early childhood, which have lowered the pain threshold.

Prior painful events are learning events that will influence interpretations of any new event and how it is handled by the adolescent or family. Early influences on the psychological or social development of the adolescent will influence coping and parental behaviours. Additionally, it is important to understand the details of the current pain, how it is managed, what precipitates it, and what maintains it. This preparation provides for a case formulation.

This chapter also presents a preliminary phase of a cognitive behavioural treatment (CBT) programme. That is, the education of the adolescent and family on how pain works in the body and the non-pharmacological influences on it. As discussed in the Introduction, education is a standard accepted practice in cognitive behavioural therapy and there is evidence that education brings positive changes in physical outcomes in adults with chronic pain.[1]

Chapter 2 continues this preliminary education work by addressing medical matters that arise from the medical path travelled by the family, the diagnosis, and their subsequent beliefs which impact on attitudes to therapy. In the adult population with chronic pain, patients' beliefs about the nature of their pain predict the outcomes in function.[2]

In a pain-education session it is possible to discuss pain resulting from damage or harm; what other pain is, and what influences pain other than medication.

Health professionals significantly underestimate the patient's ability to understand the concepts in pain education.[3] However, given that the beliefs of the adolescent or adult underpin the success of outcomes, education would seem a necessary part of treatment. Allied health therapists are ideally placed to assist in clarifying for the adolescent and family their understanding of the medical status.

Assessment

A solo therapist may be the only practitioner available to treat an adolescent with a number of issues that contribute to a multifactorial pain picture. Previous therapists may have had a single focus in therapy, e.g. exercise for a painful limb, or counselling for self-esteem or school issues. It is advantageous for a solo therapist to assess all aspects that may impact on the adolescent and their family. In this way they can engage other appropriate therapists, and they are also more likely to understand why previous therapies may have stalled.

Therapists need to ask themselves whether the questions asked will assist with their case formulation or their treatment. It is important that the adolescent and family understand the purpose of questions that may otherwise appear to be irrelevant or prying. A brief explanation of the biopsychosocial model may give tacit permission to ask some more difficult or personal questions. Some of the directions of questions suggested below may not be relevant for each adolescent. What to leave out and what to include is a matter of clinical judgement on the part of the assessor.

Information obtained in the assessment suggested below may alert the treating therapist to some of the 'yellow flags' identified throughout this book (described in the Introduction). As the narrative unfolds, it is often apparent what questions to omit and what to be more interested in.

> •*Empathy for the difficulties and feelings experienced by the family is essential.*•

Preparation

It is useful to explain the purpose of the assessment and to indicate to the adolescent and family that some questions may not seem to concern pain. Explain that a complete picture of lifestyle and personal history is important because pain can affect, and be affected by, so many areas of a person's life. It may also be useful to ask if anyone has implied that the pain is 'all in the head' or if they have felt that others doubted the pain. Give assurances that you believe the pain is real and that at a later time you can give some explanation of how pain works in the body. (No one comes to treatment for fun!)

If the adolescent or parents are very concerned that the pain is physical, any questions about mood or family background may be perceived by them as intrusive and irrelevant. Again, an empathetic response acknowledging their feelings and a discussion about their success so far with 'physical' treatment may help. Give them time to digest the significance of that discussion, possibly alerting them to the existence of the 'fat file' syndrome. (It may be that the family are not ready to consider any explanation other than a physical one at this time. They may not be ready for a biopsychosocial model of treatment at this time.)

The 'fat file' is the thick medical file in hospitals or surgeries which is a common occurrence in the case of chronic or persistent pain. 'Fat files' exist because people understandably seeking an answer or a cure, visit several doctors, each offering multiple tests and a different interpretation. The trouble with going to many specialists is that it frequently creates confusion and frustration. In the meantime, the life of the adolescent and family remains in limbo. Frequently the actions needed to regain their life are ultimately unchanged by their experience of the medical merry-go-round. It is important to acknowledge that more than one opinion may be necessary but it is advisable to accept the majority opinion rather than to seek a preferred answer.

It is important when hearing the adolescent's story that the areas described below are not pursued in a mechanical fashion simply for the sake of getting 'the facts', but that they arise from empathetic interest and an understanding of why the question may be relevant to the case formulation and treatment.

Case formulation

A complete case formulation may not be possible from a single assessment. A developmental history may be required if there is an indication of significant events or difficulties in early infancy. Additional information may be required from schools or treating practitioners to clarify details of academic performance or medical history.

The following grid can be helpful in understanding the multiple factors that may be contributing. Identifying processes, triggers, reinforcers and maintainers can assist in conceptualising the learning process that has occurred for the adolescent.

Initial assessment

Personal details
- What is the name, age, contact details and availability of the adolescent?

Note
+ Include distance and manner of travel to place of treatment as ease and availability will affect treatment schedules.

Family structure
- Who lives at home, and what are their names, ages and activities or occupations?
- What are the circumstances and dates of any marital separation?
- What is the frequency and nature of any access to the separated parent?
- What are the parents' occupations?
- How do the parents' occupations impact on the domestic timetable?
- Are any family members ill or do any have pain?

Note
+ These questions may indicate family stresses or significant family dynamics (include the time commitments of parental occupations).

Medical history
- What is the diagnosis and who made it?
- Are there other sources of information they have sought other than doctors?

⊃ Are they happy with this diagnosis or do they feel more tests or other opinions should be sought?
⊃ What investigations and treatments have occurred so far? Were they successful?

Notes
✦ Include medications and current treatment regime.
✦ Ask what the source of any information is (e.g. a neighbour may have died of cancer).
✦ Ask to see any printed matter or internet information they have consulted as this can be misleading or unbalanced.
✦ Make sense of the timeline of the history and look for any 'meaning' for the adolescent or parents associated with the event by understanding the context in which the pain occurred, i.e. who was there and what action was taken by whom; what else was happening in the family at the time, etc. This may reveal anything from a public humiliation to complex issues associated with compensation claims or issues associated with emotional attachment.

Lifestyle changes and function
⊃ Have they changed anything in order to try to control the pain?
⊃ What have they done to try to control the pain?
⊃ Has it worked?
⊃ How has the pain affected their lifestyle?
⊃ What activities have been stopped?
⊃ For how long can they sit, stand, walk and run?
⊃ How many stairs can they climb and how frequently are they required to climb them in a day or week?
⊃ How often and for how long do they lie down in the day?
⊃ How has this impacted on family members and family activities?
⊃ How are they sleeping?

Note
✦ Ask for details about sleep, e.g. time of going to bed; place of sleeping; activities prior to sleep; time to initiate sleep; frequency and reasons for waking; actions taken and by whom if waking during the night; time of waking in the morning; feeling state on waking.

⊃ How is their health generally?
⊃ Has their diet or weight changed?

Notes
✦ If weight is an issue, include recent gains or losses – this may need verifying from another source.
✦ Ask for a typical day's food and drink schedule, especially for adolescents with chronic daily headache.

✦ Enquire about other health issues, such as earlier illnesses, current chronic illnesses, or operations.

Personal interests and activities
➲ What do they do on weekends?
➲ What is their favourite activity?
➲ What do they hope to do when they are grown up?

Schooling
➲ What school do they go to?
➲ What year are they in?
➲ Have they been to other schools in the past? When?
➲ What were the reasons for change?
➲ Do they like school?
➲ What do they like/not like about school?
➲ What are their major difficulties at school?
➲ What are their friendships? Have they been bullied?
➲ When and what happened at that time?
➲ How much school has been missed? Why?
➲ Do they currently achieve a full day at school?
➲ If not, what is the process of deciding to not go, or to leave early?
➲ In what way does pain interfere?
➲ Are they able to keep up with any friends?
➲ How are they going academically in relation to their peers?
➲ How do they get to and from school and how long does it take?
➲ Whom would they prefer to nominate as their contact person?

Notes
✦ Obtain permission from the parent and adolescent to make contact with their nominated contact person. It is necessary to explain that you (the therapist) can then work with the school on any of the problems identified by them. An idea of what is preventing school attendance may emerge during discussion. Pursue avenues as they arise during discussion, e.g. bullying; teacher relations; discrepancies between attendance, academic performance and vocational aspirations; social isolation/rejection from peers, etc.
✦ In asking about how pain interferes, attempt to understand details around length of concentration, behaviour of the adolescent and the behaviour of the teacher or school at that time. It may be school policy that causes the adolescent to be sent home.

Parent and child relations
➲ Is the adolescent or parent a worrier?
➲ Is there conflict in the family?
➲ Is there anyone in the family who also has pain or is sick?

Notes
+ It may not be necessary or appropriate to ask these questions especially if there is an assessment from a psychologist. If there is no psychologist's assessment, some indication of how the family functions is necessary as it is in this context that any treatment occurs for the adolescent.
+ It may be appropriate to ask if the parents would like to be seen separately as there may be things they wish to discuss without their child present, either initially or later. Much information can be gained by observing body language and family interactions with parents and adolescent together (main speaker, chair position, physical contact and gaze during the interview are important, e.g. a father sitting further away while mother and child touch or engage constantly – this is frequently the case with an enmeshed mother and child).
+ It can be necessary to direct questions to specific members who are silent or to ask a mother to allow the adolescent to answer. This can be done by simply saying, 'I would like to hear X's story please.'
+ It can be useful to ask for the adolescent's view of themselves and how the parent sees them. Are they a worrier? Has their mood been affected? What have the parents noticed has changed in their child/themselves?
+ Explore any illnesses within the family as these may affect learning for the adolescent.

Expected outcome
➲ What would they like to have as an outcome of treatment?

Notes
+ The answer to this question can be illuminating, even surprising. Answers are always useful as a basis for further discussion.
+ Ask each family member what they expect from attending therapy. This question identifies the reality of their expectations and is the basis for a later discussion about direction and likely outcomes.
+ Answers may alert the therapist to unrealistic expectations such as removal of pain.

Pain history
➲ The modified Eland diagram, depicted in Figure 1.1, is a useful tool to help an adolescent describe their pain.
➲ Show the adolescent the picture of the body.
➲ Ask the adolescent to choose three coloured pencils; indicate that they may not need to use all three.
➲ Choose the colour they want to show their worst pain. Colour the box marked 'severe' pain with this colour, then use the same colour to shade where this worst pain is in the body in the picture. It can be in more than one place.

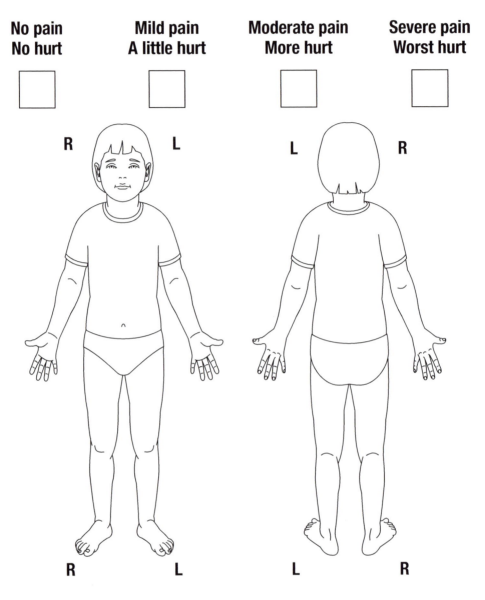

No pain
No hurt

Mild pain
A little hurt

Moderate pain
More hurt

Severe pain
Worst hurt

FIGURE 1.1 Modified Eland diagram

⊃ If there is an area or areas that also have pain but less severe, choose a different colour for the box for 'moderate pain' and shade these areas on the body.

⊃ Do the same with a third colour in the box marked 'mild pain'.

⊃ The last box stays white to show where there is no pain on the body.

Note

✦ If the adolescent has difficulty comprehending instructions break the task down, by issuing them with just one coloured pencil at a time.

✦ Once this has been completed, use the completed figure to ask them to describe each pain (ask for a descriptive word), when it occurs and whether it is constant or fluctuating. It is useful to note this on the figure.

✦ Choose the worst pain identified in the figure and ask the following questions regarding:

pain patterns in a day or week

when is pain worst

pain levels 0–10 (where 10 is the worst imaginable)

pain now

pain in last month   least

                                 average

                                 worst

frequency of the worst pain in the last month

length of pain flare-up (minutes, hours, days)

What makes it better? What do you do for yourself, what do others do for you? (i.e. coping behaviours)

What makes pain worse?

How do others know that the pain is there?

Physical assessment

⊃ A thorough physical assessment by a physiotherapist or doctor is necessary, if this is not already documented. Such an assessment must pay particular attention to strength, co-ordination or flexibility that impact on pain or that are a secondary result of guarding or longstanding immobility.

Note

✦ Notice inconsistencies of reportage, catastrophising language.

The process of the biopsychosocial assessment will give a broad picture of the pain as it is now and the factors that have contributed to the current pattern and meaning.

Table 1.1 below summarises common issues, which may become evident during assessment. It is useful as it indicates the influence of developmental history and the learning processes associated with pain.

TABLE 1.1 Examples of factors influencing pain

	PREDISPOSING	PRECIPITATING	MAINTAINING
Biological	Repeated experiences of pain in infancy lowering pain thresholds. Genetic predisposition to low pain threshold. Sleep problems.	An injury or illness. Medical intervention (surgery or other). Immobilisation and consequent loss of fitness. Fatigue.	Poor fitness levels leading to increased pain on movement and withdrawal from activity. Negative effect and low energy levels.
Psychological	Maternal illness leading to poor attachment. Marital disharmony. Familial trait of anxiety or avoidant coping. Maternal separation issues. Low IQ, Asperger's syndrome. Trauma or loss in family. Early schema of victimhood/helplessness/hopelessness/perfection. 'Precious' only child or last child. Low self-esteem. Inability to set boundaries on behaviours/Poor emotional regulation. Assumption of a sick role.	Emotional independence required in transition from primary to secondary school – stalled individuation. Bullying. Erratic school attendance initiating academic crisis. High academic expectations leading to anxiety, anger, depression. Parental fear of damage to child.	Deprivation of opportunities for coping skills (due to parental protectiveness). School absenteeism and lack of school support causing lag in learning. Ongoing reinforcement of avoidant responses by social withdrawal. Unhelpful family stories. Excessive attention to pain.
Social	Social isolation due to family culture or distance. A family culture of illness or disability. Frequent family moves disrupting schooling. Absence of siblings that would challenge or moderate behaviours.	Social isolation at school due to not keeping up with peers' activities. No adequate bullying policy at school. Deprivation of social skills due to school absences. Absence of challenges by peers.	Parental acceptance of ongoing isolation.

Pain education

The following is an outline of key considerations in explaining the mechanisms of pain to adolescents, with a discussion of session format.

Preparation for pain education

The therapist should outline for the family at the beginning of the session that the aim of this information is to empower them so that they can make up their own minds. It is a forum for them to hear in layperson's language as best as possible what is known about pain and what influences it. They do not have to remember any details in particular, but some handouts may help them recall the gist of the information later. Offer to explore any information with them but emphasise that although it is in the form of general facts, as we know them at this time, they may find themselves interpreting the information according to their circumstances. They can choose to explore this as the session continues. The information may also serve to explain why several health professions may become involved and why so many other aspects, other than the management of physical experience of pain, are dealt with in the management of persistent pain. The multiplicity of factors that influence pain reflects the physiology of pain in the body.

Who should be there?

Usually, it is useful to have significant family members in the same session as a discussion between members may clarify and identify behaviours around pain. However, it may be judged appropriate for the individuating adolescent to be seen separately when the adolescent has a desire for privacy that is thwarted because the parent constantly intervenes. Seeing the adolescent separately may also be appropriate if the adolescent does not understand or is unwilling to take responsibility, since the session can be used to present to them that their active participation is what is required and is more important than that of parents or health practitioners.

It may be useful to have a separate session with parents if there is the possibility of parents feeling challenged or upset by the information. A session with the parents alone allows them to speak freely. This can be particularly so when there is a discrepancy between the parents' committed belief in the adolescent's 'illness' and what has been diagnosed, or if they feel the information presented calls into question their interpretation of their adolescent's behaviour.

Designing and managing a session

Following thorough history taking, assessment and case formulation, it will be apparent that some areas of an education session will be more significant than others for an individual, so the focus of sessions will vary considerably. Extra time and detail may be spent on relevant areas to stimulate discussion in the context of the individual's history.

Although the facts of a session are presented as general facts of physiology, parents and adolescents tend to personalise their application and draw inferences for their situation. In this way the therapist can discuss areas that are likely to be addressed in intervention. Examples are a more detailed description of social learning theory in a family where there are multiple members with pain, or a family exhibiting fear-avoidance. A discussion may be possible about how family members know when others are in pain. This discussion lends itself to identifying those pain behaviours that may be legitimately addressed in treatment sessions. 'Dos and don'ts' (*see* Chapter 8) are much more easily accepted. Asking questions of the adolescent or parent throughout the education session is essential in order to engage them, to enable them to think through and problem solve for themselves, and to clarify their understanding of pain. This is likely to be the first time they have had the opportunity to do this.

Additionally, education may be a form of assessment of the parent's readiness for acceptance of therapy. The information that links the thinking plus learning processes with emotions and the experience of pain challenges the commonly held paradigm of pain as purely a manifestation of physical damage. The material presented in an education session and which invites acceptance of psychological intervention is a challenge that the parent may not be prepared to accept. Even if a physical programme of rehabilitation is undertaken, it may also not succeed due to the underlying parent and family dynamic that maintains the child's illness behaviour.

Discussion requires sensitivity to gauge the degree of threat posed to, and openness to change in members of the family. The therapist must emphasise that the information is general and applies to everybody and that there is no need for the parents to personalise their response. They may take time to digest it and they may want to discuss it later. They may decide this is true for others but not for them. A common response to feeling challenged is to react with anger; therefore, it is important to ask how the session has affected the adolescent or family members, thus allowing for any anger to be expressed. If the session has been upsetting it is important to acknowledge this and to make a time to listen to their responses at the earliest possible time following the session.

Anatomy of a session

The following is an outline of the content of a pain-education session. It is presented in question form, with each question followed by a discussion of common responses and issues that arise. It may happen that the session becomes sidetracked by an in-depth discussion on a particular area of interest, and this must be followed through. The adolescent's or parent's response may need to be added to, modified, or corrected by the therapist. The therapist needs to check for understanding during the session and it is important to encourage questions or clarification as needed throughout.

> *Therapist asks the adolescent:* 'What would happen if there was no pain?'
>
> *An adolescent's common answer:* 'It would be great because I could do whatever I want!'
>
> *Therapist's elaboration:* 'First think what would happen if people never had pain. At first it sounds great, but if you think about it, this would mean we would keep hurting ourselves without even realising. Pain is like our body's own 'alarm system' that warns us when there is injury or when injury is likely to occur. This is

important because it lets us know what is happening, and can stop further injury. For example, if you touch a hot stove, pain tells you that it is too hot, so your instant reaction is to take your hand away so that it doesn't get burnt. At that time you may show pain by crying out. You may also be able to choose not to show this pain behaviour if you were hiding from someone. In other words you could still have the pain and not show it. Afterwards, if your hand still hurt because you may have developed a blister, this would be pain due to damage to the skin that would cause you to seek ointment or a bandage. You can see from this that you must think about pain when it happens: do I cry out, do I need a bandage or a doctor? Your pain system can also alert you if you stretch a muscle too far, so that you don't tear it. Pain is a powerful survival mechanism that is designed to interrupt whatever you are doing. It demands first priority of your attention. It is your friend that stops you from cooking your hand without knowing it! It is designed to be very powerful. For this reason it is not possible to expect to completely ignore pain or distract yourself. If you don't understand whether there is damage, it is natural to feel 'alarmed', like when you hear a fire alarm. It's only when you know it's a false alarm that you can go back to what you are doing. Pain makes you vigilant, it doesn't want you to forget about it and it strongly puts you off continuing whatever action you were doing when it happens. In this, it can be your foe, because it can become your boss! It is the most powerfully unpleasant sense we have so it is natural to want to avoid it.'

Therapist: 'What have you been doing to avoid pain? Has it worked? Do you think it's possible for a person to never have pain, to always avoid it?'

[Discuss how the adolescent employs avoidance activities so that these can be addressed at a later date.]

Therapist: 'Do you feel your pain has become the boss, has it has taken you over now? Discuss in what way this has happened.'

Therapist: 'What have you been told about your pain/diagnosis?'

[There are many responses to this question, so it is important to clarify any misunderstandings the person might have, and to begin to fill in the gaps in their knowledge of their diagnosis (*see* Chapter 2). You may assist them to source good information. They may have consulted the internet and encountered chat rooms that give misleading emphasis to a diagnosis. Hypothesise with the adolescent and family around possible explanations, based on the best possible information. Information may come from handouts, the doctor, physiotherapist, osteopath and other alternative therapists. Offer to seek further clarification on their behalf. Stress the fact that you believe that they are experiencing real pain. If no diagnosis is clear and there are conflicting views, offer a way forward, 'Shall we try this . . . or this . . .? Which is most likely to lead to moving forward?' 'How will you know whether you have moved forward?' Avoid a lengthy discussion on this by offering a later session on identifying their own goals.

Therapist: 'Do you feel that all medical issues have been explored?'

Common answers: 'No, they haven't done an MRI . . . etc. . . . and I would like that to be done' or 'One doctor said X and another said Y . . .'

[It may be helpful to describe how a diagnosis is arrived at and why an MRI may not have been an appropriate test. Chapter 2 deals with this in more detail.]

Therapist: 'What have you been taught about nerves?'

'Did you know we have two nervous systems, one that we are conscious of, like when we are touched or when we move? This is called the sensory-motor system. The other system is the autonomic system – it sounds a little like 'automatic'. This system works without us having to consciously make it happen. It governs all the automatic responses in the body, like sweating when nervous or too hot, increasing blood supply for healing, digesting your food, maintaining your heart beat and breathing. All of these happen without you having to remember to do it! We will talk about how these two systems work together later.'

[Explore what they already understand, and fill in the gaps.]

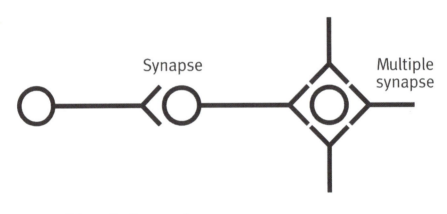

FIGURE 1.2 Schematic diagram of a nerve

'Nerves are like our body's own electrical wires that send electrical messages around the body. Nerves have two endings, like an extension cord so that one nerve can connect with the next one. There are millions of these connections in the body and brain. There is a gap in between one nerve and the next. Messages can pass or be stopped at the connection (synapse), depending on what type of chemicals (neurotransmitters) have been released into the space at the synapse, between one nerve and another. We will talk more about these chemicals later.'

'We have sensory nerve endings (receptors) in our body that can respond to different stimuli, such as touch, temperature, pressure, stretch, position and movement. etc. These give us useful information about what is happening both inside and outside our body. Some receptors pick up information from outside our body so we know what things feel like – whether they are hot/cold, sharp/

smooth, soft/hard, etc. Others tell us about what happens inside our body and in our muscles. If you close your eyes and move your arm above your head you will still know exactly where it is in space, because of messages from these position and movement receptors. If I touch your arm, you know that I have touched your arm because a sensory nerve has sent a message to your brain.'

Therapist: 'What happens when we feel pain?'

'Receptors (at the end of nerve) that pick up normal sensations are the same ones that can register pain. Normal 'feeling-type' sensory messages can become pain messages if receptors are stimulated to the level of what we call a 'pain threshold'. This is because sensory receptors have what we call a 'pain threshold'. Everyone will have a slightly different pain threshold. Your pain threshold is the point where that hot stove, sharp object or tight muscle or stretched joint becomes painful. (You may say 'ouch' quicker or slower than another person.)'

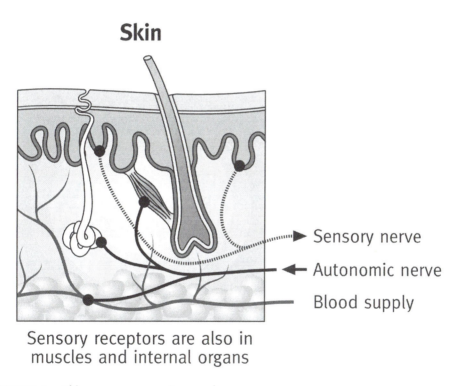

Skin

Sensory nerve

Autonomic nerve

Blood supply

Sensory receptors are also in muscles and internal organs

FIGURE 1.3 Skin, sensory receptors and nerves

'For these sensory nerves to reach the brain, they first have to travel to the spinal cord, which is a big bundle of little nerves travelling together, like a big rope. The spinal cord travels through the centre of the bones (vertebrae) in your spine.'

'Can you feel those bones in your back?'

*•If someone cuts the spinal cord they can't move or feel anything
below that point, i.e. they become quadriplegic or paraplegic.•*

'In the spinal cord, the sensory nerve connects with another nerve which carries
the message all the way to the brain.'

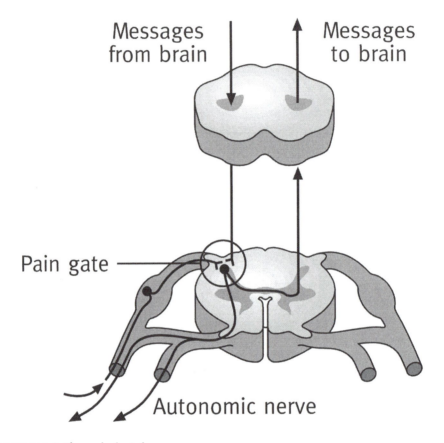

FIGURE 1.4 The pain 'gate'

Therapist: 'What happens in the brain?'

'Firstly, we may think of our bodies – including our brain – as somehow
complete or fixed. Actually, all our cells, including nerves, are constantly changing.
When we learn something new, a new connection is made in the brain by a nerve.
If we want to improve at an activity, we focus our mind on it and concentrate. In
this way, we are able to establish permanent new pathways in the brain. Whatever
we focus on and repeat we get better at, generally speaking. The same thing can
happen around pain. Let me explain.'

'All sensory nerve messages end up in a part of the brain called the sensory
cortex, which is a 'body map' that contains the nerve endings coming from all our

different body parts. There is an area in your brain that represents your hand, your leg, your nose, etc. You know that I touched your arm and not your leg because of the nerve ends up in the area corresponding to your arm. We have more sensory receptors in certain parts of our body than in others, because we need them to be more sensitive (e.g. hands, lips). Therefore there is a bigger part of the brain for these areas.' (*See* Figure 1.2.)

Researchers have found these nerve endings can actually sprout out into the surrounding areas, making it larger and creating greater sensitivity to pain. This can happen when we focus on pain or use strong language about pain ('it feels like a hot poker', 'it's the worst pain ever' – we call this 'catastrophising').

'So although we believe the pain is there, we may ask you not to talk about it, or to find other language to describe your pain. For the same reason we ask that your family and friends don't ask about your pain.'

'Not asking about pain can be a hard thing for mums and dads but remember the mind is like sunlight, wherever it shines is the part that grows, so, although the pain is there, let's put it in the shadow so it won't grow. It is likely that the pain will always interrupt and want the person with pain to focus on it but if you are doing what matters to you, you can choose to keep your focus on that. Of course it is important to tell parents when it is necessary, if there is a change or if you have injured yourself.'

'We can talk about how to do this later because we know this may seem difficult but there are things to learn that will help.'

Therapist: 'The brain is very active when we feel pain!'

'Researchers have shown this by asking people to volunteer to experience pain (for example, students have been asked to put their hands into very cold water until it is painful, and then a functional MRI of their brain is performed to see which parts are working at that moment of pain.'

'In the brain, there are many areas involved when we feel pain. Three important areas are the frontal lobe, the limbic system and the thalamus.'

'These brain areas 'talk' to one another. This is where pain is 'perceived': the brain generates the experience of the body.'

[Each of the following areas may be expanded upon according to individual needs/issues.]

Therapist: 'Remember how when we get pain we think about it?'

'The frontal lobe is the part of the brain behind our forehead. In humans this part of the brain (as well as other parts of the cortex which we don't necessarily need to discuss today, i.e. parietal, occipital and temporal lobes) has developed to be very large. The frontal lobes are responsible for thinking, problem solving and learning. Of course we rely on our memories to be able to recall what we

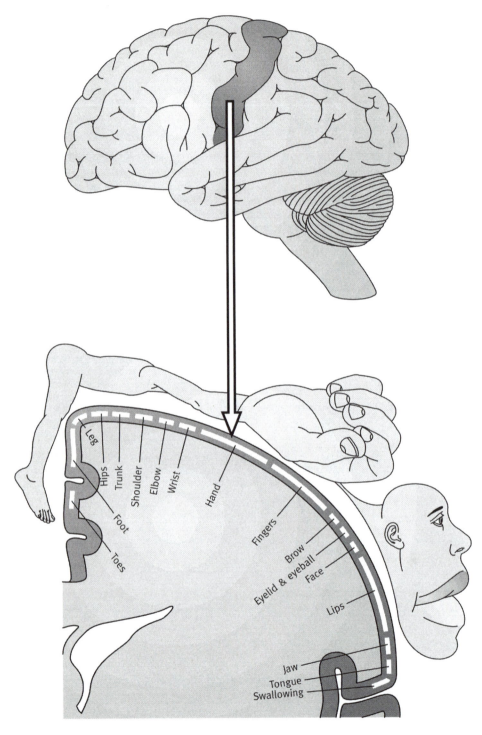

FIGURE 1.5 Sensory cortex

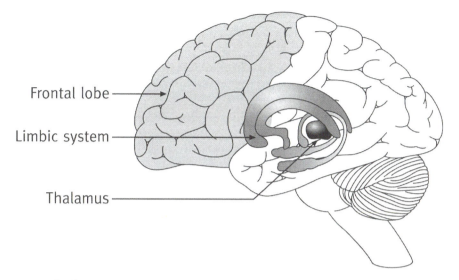

Frontal lobe

Limbic system

Thalamus

FIGURE 1.6 The brain

have learned. The frontal lobes are a complex matrix or web of trillions of nerve connections and multiple synapses we spoke of before, which have been built up over our life's learning. It is the seat of what we would call our unique personality.'

•If someone has a head injury to their forebrain, they will often have problems with memory and changes in their personality. This is because they have lost some of their accumulated learning. They may not remember what behaviour is appropriate in social situations.•

'If you think about it, it is natural to think about pain. Remember, it is about survival, and you need to think about how you will stop it happening again. Surviving is how we got to be smart! You need to decide which path of action to take, in order to survive. When we experience pain, we relate it to our previous experiences of pain and how we dealt with that pain. These experiences are unique to each individual. Depending on our experiences, we then problem-solve over what to do next, e.g. 'Last time the pain was this bad it lasted for weeks, so maybe it will this time as well.' 'What my mum does is X, so I will do that too.'

Your individual experiences and ideas of pain are likely to be different from mine, because you have different experiences of pain and your upbringing is different from mine – you have different stories to tell about pain.'

'This means that sometimes we need to look at what you think about pain and how you may have learned it and whether your problem solving is working.'

•Pavlov, a Russian scientist, discovered that you can condition animals to keep doing the same thing if you reward them. He trained dogs to salivate (autonomic nervous system response) whenever a bell rang. He did this by first giving them food every time the bell rang. He also learned that the dogs would keep on salivating even when no food came. It took a long time for the dogs to stop salivating after the food supply stopped. After the dogs stopped salivating, if food was reintroduced again with the bell even only once, the dogs instantly resumed the same behaviour as at the beginning. This was something they 'learned'. We have similar mechanisms that trigger thoughts or behaviours in us.•

'Also stored in this area is the memory of the context in which pain happens. For example, a man who lost his arm in war while saving his best friend will have a different response to that pain than someone who lost their arm because their boss didn't put a guard on a machine. The worker will blame the boss, thinking, 'It's his fault' and he is likely to feel angry. Thoughts and emotions work together – we don't usually have an emotion without a thought behind it. We feel angry for a reason. It might be a silly or false reason but it is our thought and we believe it. Scientists (neurophysiologists) have shown this association with MRIs. This leads us to the other area mentioned, the area responsible for our emotions.'

[Refer to Figure 1.6.]

'Our emotions happen in a part of the brain called the limbic system.'

Therapist: 'Have you noticed particular feelings or emotions that you have when you are in pain? Anger, frustration, sadness or worry?'

[Prompt the adolescent to explore their own feelings around pain, and then fill in the gaps from the explanation below. It can be common for some adolescents not to immediately recognise their thoughts or feelings.]

'These are common feelings people have when they have pain. You might be frustrated or cross when you can't do what you want, or if you think it is not fair when bad things happen to you, but not to your friends. Another emotion is fear, or feeling scared, worried, nervous or anxious. You might be anxious because you think that you have damaged yourself or that something bad might happen again. You might also feel sad. You tend to feel sad when you have lost something – this might be losing your dog, your friends, your lifestyle, or the ability to play your favourite sport. You might feel unhappy or depressed because you think you have to stop to avoid the pain. Again, notice that the emotion and thought go together, we don't usually have a feeling or emotion for no reason. An emotion is accompanied by a thought. We may not even be aware of what that thought is, sometimes we can only find our thoughts after we look more closely at our feelings, these will lead us back to what we are thinking. We can even have an argument with ourselves about whether we want that thought! More on that later.'

'Do you recognise any of these feelings as those that you have?'

'How can you tell in your body when you are scared or angry? What is your body doing when you get a big fright?'

[Elaborate on sensations that come with fear or anxiety – a thumping heart; breath held in and up in the upper chest; sensations of tightness in chest or stomach; nausea; faintness or dizziness (blood pressure changes). Identify all of these as responses of the autonomic nervous system and the release of adrenalin.]

'All those sensations and changes in your body we have just talked about are the work or effect of activity in the autonomic nervous system that we spoke of before.'

Therapist: 'Do you know what a gland is?'

'A gland is another means of sending messages throughout the body. We talked about nerves that send electrical messages. Glands manufacture and send chemical messages. These chemicals can either help or hinder the lessening of the feeling of pain. The autonomic nervous system has a control station called the thalamus, the third important area we identified earlier. The thalamus tells other glands to release certain hormones/chemicals into the body.'

'Remember, the autonomic nervous system is the "effective" nervous system that we talked of before, that sends messages out to the body to get it do things like sweat, salivate, heal when we damage ourselves, digest food, go to the toilet, etc.'

[This may be a good point to describe the healing process, in more detail, for adolescents diagnosed with CRPS. In particular, the swelling, colour and temperature changes and the heightened sensitivity to pain on touch or movement, all of which are initiated by the autonomic nervous system. (*See* Chapter 2 for more detail – refer to diagram of the skin.)]

'Glands release a chemical 'soup' such as adrenalin into the body, which cause these reactions to occur. There are different 'soup' recipes for different jobs. We all have our own recipe for pain killers, called endorphins. These are just like our own Panadol. Have you heard of adrenalin? What do you think it does, when does it happen and what does it feel like in your body? Have you ever had a fright?'

'If you think back to the types of feeling you might have when you are in pain, you can think of some of the reactions that happen in your body so you know you are afraid or angry. When we feel afraid or angry, our heart beats really fast, our muscles get tense, and our breathing becomes fast and shallow, sometimes we hold our breath with fright or anger.'

[If there is little recognition of these feeling states, get the adolescent to act out being angry or afraid, ask what they would have to do to look angry or afraid.]

Therapist: 'How do these three different areas contribute to the pain experience?'

'When we think about pain and relate it to past experiences and memories of pain and our learning around pain, this often leads to an emotional response. These emotions cause chemicals to be released which cause our body to react. For example, a girl might have knee pain, and start thinking about how sore it is, and how last time it was sore it was a long time before the pain went away, and then one bad thing after another followed. These thoughts make her start to feel sad and worried that maybe the pain will never go away. She may not notice it, but because she is worried, her breathing changes and she becomes very tense somewhere in her body. Her pain is likely to feel worse. This is because her thoughts and emotions have produced a chemical soup and the message is sent downwards from the thalamus, where the incoming message enters the spinal cord. The adrenalin helps the pain message to jump quickly and easily across from the incoming nerve to the upward nerve in the spinal cord so the pain is continued and increased. The chemical message from the thalamus has 'opened' the pain gate at the spinal cord.'

[Refer to Figure 1.4.]

'Have you noticed this pain increase in yourself when you are tense? Tension may occur with other events in your life as well. What happened? Being able to notice this is the beginning of being able to do things to help yourself.'

Therapist: 'So how can we influence our pain?'

'When the pain gate is 'open', pain messages are free to travel all the way to the brain. If the pain gate can start to be 'closed', then the pain messages will have a harder time getting all the way to the brain.

'Sometimes people have persistent pain, where the pain messages are still being sent even with no potential or actual tissue injury. This might be thought of as your nervous system becoming sensitised to pain – like a system with a volume control, where your system is amplifying the incoming pain messages.'

Therapist: 'How do we close the pain gate?'

'We can help close pain gate by releasing another type of chemical 'soup', called endorphins, rather than adrenalin. Endorphins contain the body's natural pain-killers. They are called opioids. (Have you heard of morphine? That is an opioid.)'

[The following may need modification according to the cognitive abilities of parents and adolescents. The issues suggesting reinforcement of pain within the family may be unsuitable to be presented – certainly initially – if there is doubt as to the receptiveness of the parents to such information or until some trust has been established.]

'A fourth area already understood as significant in people with addictions has only recently been discovered to be significant in the study of pain. MRIs have shown that this area is stimulated by noxious pain messages from the body and also by the prospect of reward. As primitive humans it would have made us choose between competing powerful motivations, e.g. whether to continue hunting for food (the high value reward) in order not to starve even though we were wounded and in pain (the noxious stimulus) with high motivation to avoid it. It is the place in the brain where we make instantaneous (unconscious) choices about whether to respond to the noxious (painful) stimulus or whether there are competing high-value stimuli that are likely to bring other rewards (food to avoid starvation). If the latter is the choice, opioids (our natural pain killers) are released and less pain is experienced. This is the likely explanation for sports people being able to continue to play the game despite having torn ligaments, or soldiers at war able to fight on despite injury. Here, there is a primitive competition between motivations. Remember how we discussed the fact that the response to pain is a primitive one about survival (i.e. to stop activity because of damage)? These footballers were so highly motivated by the rewards of kicking goals that this motivation and the prospect of reward outdid the survival motivation; they chose to ignore the pain and play on. It may also explain why, when there are significant rewards associated in the family environment (and therefore release of opioids), it is very hard for an adolescent to choose to do activities away from home that would diminish that reward. This is especially so if the other activities provoke anxiety. It would mean having more pain until other rewards are established. That is a hard request to make, given the primitive power of pain. It is, however, what we need to do. We need to find what you value and what motivates you, i.e. activities which are rewarding for you.'

'Do you remember describing what it felt like in your body when you are worried or fearful; tense, tight or jumpy muscles, fast breathing or breath held in upper chest, fast heart beat? The opposite is slow, deep-down breathing, relaxed, soft muscles, slow heart beat, etc. These reactions are what happen when you are relaxed and the body has released endorphins. Endorphins are the chemical 'soup' that happens when you are laughing, having fun and are relaxed; this is where you find your natural pain killers. So part of what we do is to find out how to increase the fun and to teach you skills that will purposely relax you. We can't change our heart beat or sweating, but we can change our breathing which in turn affects the body. We can learn to do this with breathing techniques.'

'Have you ever done meditation or relaxation before?'

[Ask the child for their experience and affirm the intention to do it differently if the experience was negative, and delay discussion till later (*see* Chapter 6).]

Therapist: 'The treatment sessions to follow are based on what influences pain – as we have just talked about!'

'What we do in the pain clinic is to find as many ways of getting your body to release these natural pain killers, so you can have the rewards of a full life.'

'This means finding what motivates you, getting involved in activities that will engage your attention so there is no focus on pain, learning relaxation techniques and looking at the thought/emotions circuit that may be influencing the pain gate.'

(*See* www.radcliffe-oxford.com/adolescentpain for handout of the pain system and what opens and closes the pain gate.)

Other information to discuss as need arises:
Hurt versus harm

> *Therapist:* 'It is important to understand that sometimes when you feel pain it will mean there is harm or potential for harm, but at other times you can feel pain which may be a reaction to stretch or some other stimuli that will not actually cause you any damage. This can happen for a variety of reasons.'
>
> [Explore possibilities relevant to the individual. Check their understanding of whether their pain is hurt or harm and why – this may link in with their diagnosis, conflicting advice from others, or ignorance about anatomy, physiology or body mechanics, etc.]

Overdoing versus underdoing

> *Therapist:* 'It is important to pace your activities, and gradually get yourself back into things one step at a time. It is important to understand what the right amount of activity is for you. Are you the sort of person that keeps going even when you know you have reached your limit? Let's talk more about this later.'

Deconditioning

> *Therapist:* 'Being unfit can cause feelings of discomfort and pain when new exercise first begins. For instance, if I were to go for a long run now I would probably hurt afterwards. This is not because I have injured myself, but just because my muscles have been stretched and used in a way I am not used to.'
>
> 'Because you have had longstanding pain it is possible to interpret this sort of stretch as part of an earlier experience of pain due to injury.'

New learning and old (*see also* Chapter 5)

> *Therapist:* 'We learn in whole lot of different ways. We learn in school when we listen to facts or solve a puzzle but we also learn in other ways. Some of these we don't even notice even as they are happening. We learn from our friends and family just by watching and imitating them. This is called modelling. This is how families come to seem so alike in mannerisms or ways of doing things. This can be just the same with pain. Some families don't talk about or show their feelings and are like this about pain. Others are very demonstrative in showing they are in pain by holding sore areas, limping or crying. We can talk later about which is more helpful for you.'
>
> 'Another way we learn is that if something happens over and over, we tend to predict that it will happen again. Just like Pavlov's dogs that salivated when the bell rang. This is because the dogs have seen a pattern and an association even to the point of their body responding automatically. It takes time for this learning to change once a pattern or association has been established.'
>
> [Having presented the factors that influence the pain gate it is both logical

and reassuring to give the family and adolescent an idea of what will be done in following sessions.]

Pain management strategies

Therapist: 'Pain management strategies aim to give you a sense that there are actions that you can take that are helpful for you, so you can restore your life and put pain in the back seat rather than in the driver's seat. Research has shown that people who believe in their own ability to take effective action when having pain will actually feel less pain. These strategies are things you can do for yourself.'

Being engaged in life activities

Therapist: 'If you are very busy doing something that is important to you, you will most likely feel less pain than when you are bored. Primarily our focus will be on pursuing that chosen activity even though pain may still interrupt that focus. This will entail spending time on identifying your values and goals and on reaching a level of fitness that allows you to do them.'

Relaxation/meditation/breathing techniques

Therapist: 'Relaxation is another way of changing the pain gate. If you think about the autonomic nervous system, most of it occurs without us having any control over it. For example, we can't purposely increase our heart rate and make it beat faster or make ourselves sweat simply by thinking about it. However, one aspect which we can purposely alter is our breathing. If we can slow down our breathing and become relaxed, this affects the rest of the autonomic nervous system. This in turn can change the 'chemical soups' in our body.'

Awareness of your thinking and feelings

Therapist: 'Sometimes the things we think can be unhelpful. Remember how the thinking and emotional areas of the brain communicate with each other? Our thoughts and emotions are very closely related. Learning to become mindful of your thinking is a way to put these unpleasant thoughts and feelings in perspective and stop battling with them. If we feel happy, calm, or relaxed rather than frustrated or worried, our body will release endorphins rather than adrenalin, and this will help to close the pain gate.'

Case study: Mona

Mona was a 13-year-old girl who presented with general body pain which she believed was due to juvenile rheumatoid arthritis (JRA). At the time of assessment, this diagnosis was awaiting clarification from blood-test results. However, the consultant Rheumatologist had indicated that he felt that the symptomatology was not consistent with JRA. Mona identified herself as suffering from anxiety which, along with her pain, was exacerbated by attending school. She had not attended school for eight months. Assessment also revealed considerable family discord, with a father who was largely absent and a mother suffering post-traumatic stress. Mona was unusually able to describe how the pain saved her from facing that which she feared, i.e. school attendance. In her words, it was her 'shield'. She understood that the pain was useful to her and did not want to have an MRI as recommended, in case, like the blood test, it returned as negative to JRA.

During the education session, both Mona and her mother were able to understand pain differently. They felt that the explanation of physiology of pain acknowledged the pain as real and they were able to discuss the possibility of results negative to JRA. They were able to accept psychological assistance after understanding the relationship between pain and their psychological issues. Mona's mother described relief. Despite her own anxiety, she became committed to supporting a return-to-school programme for Mona, seeking help for herself as part of the process. The physiology of pain needed to be repeated several times for Mona who experienced considerable resistance to her return to school, citing the pain as her reason for needing to go home.

Initially, she did not want the school to know her pain was not from JRA, and she requested a special chair and cushion. Her school was contacted and strategies advised. Her return to school was programmed so that it was predictable for her and therefore less anxiety provoking. She was to attend for exactly one class at 9.00 a.m. daily. This was increased incrementally as her tolerance increased. The pain was managed with breathing techniques and behavioural strategies to be practised at school (without a special chair and cushion).

Further reading

Bayer T, Baer PE, Early C. Situational and psychophysiological factors in psychologically induced pain. *Pain*. 1991; **44**(1): 45–50.

Becerra L, Breoter HC, Wise R, *et al*. Reward circuitry activation by noxious thermal stimuli. *Neuron*. 2001; **32**: 927–46.

Field H. State-dependent opioid control of pain. *Nat Res Neurosci*. 2004; **5**: 565–75.

Field HA. Motivation-decision model of pain: the role of opioids. In: Flor H, Kalso E, Dostrovsky JO, editors. Proceedings of the 11th World Congress on Pain; 2006; Seattle: IASP Press, pp. 449–59.

Flor H. In: *Progress in Brain Research*, Vol 129. Amsterdam: Elsevier Science; 2000, pp. 313–22.

Wall PD, Melzack R. *Textbook of Pain*, 4th ed. Edinburgh: Churchill Livingstone; 1999.

References

1 Lorimer ML. Evidence for a direct relationship between cognitive and physical change during an education intervention in people with chronic low back pain. *Eur J Pain*. 2004; 8: 39–45.

2 Jensen MP, Nielson WR, Romano JM, *et al*. Patient beliefs predict patient functioning: further support for a cognitive-behavioural model of chronic pain. *Pain*. 1999; **81**: 95–104.

3 Lorimer ML. Unravelling the barriers to reconceptualisation of the problem in chronic pain: the actual and perceived ability of patients and health professionals to understand the neurophysiology. *Pain*. 2003; **4**(4): 184–9.

CHAPTER 2

Medical matters

ABOUT DIAGNOSIS, TESTS AND DISORDERS

CHAPTER SUMMARY

This chapter presents common medical journeys the family and adolescent are likely to have taken and the effect this has had on them. It outlines the difficulties of doctors and medical systems and offers suggestions for overcoming misconceptions for the family using the 'doctor as detective' metaphor to clarify the process of diagnosis. Limiting factors are discussed. Common questions asked by adolescents and families are answered. This is followed by simple explanations for use by clinicians to clarify the use of common tests and referrals to medical specialists in the continuing journey to seek clarity on medical matters. A list of conditions commonly associated with chronic pain and referred for pain management is included.

Background

Some common causes of persistent pain that present to a specialist pain-management clinic in young people are headaches, abdominal pain, arthritis, musculo-skeletal pain (fibromyalgia, strains and sprains), post-operative complications such as scarring or nerve damage, complex regional pain syndrome and pain of unknown cause. These referrals may be made by specialists after extensive investigations. Therapists in solo practice or not working in a specialised pain team need a clear understanding of the diagnosis and medical support for the programme they present to the adolescent and family.

There are areas of medicine that specialise in conditions with which pain is frequently associated. Oncology, orthopaedics, rheumatology, gynaecology and neurology are some examples, not to mention the multiple specialties involved in traumatic events. Many conditions involve periodic episodes of acute pain that are managed better by some adolescents and their families than by others. While it is not within the scope of this book to deal with acute pain or with underlying disease processes, many of the same biopsychosocial issues and management strategies may be relevant for some adolescents with these problems, and their families.

Parents who have a child with persistent pain have usually sought help from many different sources prior to seeking assistance directly for pain management. It is important for the therapist to understand any family's journey, prior to their presenting for assessment for pain management. Misconceptions about diagnosis, investigations and the roles of practitioner abound in this process. These easily lead to troublesome beliefs and emotional consequences for the adolescent and parents – with confusion, anger, frustration, disappointment, or blaming directed specifically at one practitioner, or generalised to groups or institutions. Many doctors and allied health professionals operate from a bio-medical model with pain, i.e. pain equates to damage or pathology. Having not found underlying pathology for pain within their particular area of specialty (orthopaedics, rheumatology, gastroenterology, gynaecology, etc.) doctors may infer – or directly state – that as the pain is not 'physical' it is in the 'head' of the child, i.e. it's psychological. For the adolescent experiencing the pain this is at best unbelievable as they know their pain is a very 'physical' sensation. At worst they feel insulted as it implies that they are either imagining it or pretending. In the face of disbelief from others, they may feel even more inclined to 'prove' their pain to their parent and others by increasing the outward signs of pain, i.e. displaying pain behaviour (groaning, crying, limping, etc.). This behaviour may present as inconsistent with the original diagnosis. Some health practitioners interpret this as 'manipulative' behaviour.

Doctors are usually expected to make a clear diagnosis and, if possible, cure the problem. With persistent pain, this may not happen. The neurophysiology of chronic pain is a specialist area, requiring specialist training. Doctors from specialties other than pain are unlikely to have in-depth expertise about persistent pain. Furthermore, problems can arise in the doctor–patient relationship. Doctors, after having tried to relieve their patient's pain, can interpret persistent pain in their patient as a failure, and (defensively) blame the patient. Parents can feel 'handballed' from one doctor to another and feel they are the only advocate for their child in this situation. When they exhibit solicitous behaviour towards their child it can be negatively interpreted. Parents too, can feel defensive and blamed.

The following are difficulties that can arise with doctors.

➲ They may not be good communicators and may be unable to explain clearly the complex neurophysiology of pain. They may not believe that explanations are helpful.

➲ They may be ill-informed about the neurophysiology of persistent pain.

➲ The patient relies on the knowledge of the doctor. For this reason, the patient may be guided in directions that they learn later are unhelpful in the long term, e.g. 'rest when it hurts', 'increase the medication', 'let's do more tests just in case', etc.

➲ The doctor may focus on diagnosis within their specialty. This leads to serial referrals frequently without an overall case manager to make sense of the multiple results from the patient's perspective.

➲ Doctors contradict one another and may not communicate with other treating doctors.

➲ Doctors are powerful in the holding of their knowledge; they may promise a 'cure' or a diagnosis when there is none.

Similar difficulties can arise with allied health professionals as well, including promises of cures and prolonged treatments that make no difference to the adolescent's life yet which cost the family large sums of money.

Overcoming misconceptions for the family

The therapist needs to make an appropriate clinical choice as to how much medical detail is of benefit to each adolescent and parent (remembering that clinicians consistently underestimate the capacity of their patients to understand).[1]

After the capacity of the family to comprehend and accept new information has been assessed, an exploration of what they know regarding the medical process may reveal the basis for idiosyncratic beliefs or negative emotions that are unhelpful. Clarification can assist them in changing beliefs and accepting a therapeutic process.

Parents and adolescents may:

➲ have a poor understanding of the anatomy and physiology of the body

➲ have little understanding of the way in which a diagnosis is made (i.e. based on scientific evidence and deduction)

➲ have contradictory information from different doctors or between alternative medical practitioners and doctors

➲ have misinformation from the internet or second-hand information from friends

➲ not understand the role of different medical specialties.

Doctor as detective

It can be helpful for the therapist to explain to parents and the adolescent the 'art' as well as the science of making a diagnosis so that they understand it is not guesswork and that, although rigour is applied, there are sometimes difficulties in arriving at absolute conclusions. The metaphor of 'doctors as detectives' is a useful one to explain the process to families. It can be readily understood because of the plethora of detective and crime shows on television.

It may not be necessary to provide a full explanation; however, for some interested adolescents or parents it can lessen the expectations that the medical process is perfect. The following may be a helpful explanation.

> *Therapist:* 'Doctors, like detectives are trained to read 'signs' in the body (i.e. what the doctor can find for themselves on examination). These, plus the patient's report of their experience (symptoms), are the evidence from which they deduce the disease process within the anatomy and biochemistry of the body (the pathophysiology). They name it or, in other words, make a diagnosis. The signs and symptoms are the 'evidence', from which the doctor makes an hypothesis of a diagnosis. If the hypothesis is shown to be correct (tests may be used), he has made a diagnosis. This process is called 'deduction' and is the basis of a scientific process. It is not guesswork! Doctors make the diagnosis of the underlying condition, based on the particular collection and pattern of signs and symptoms.'
>
> 'Sometimes there is more than one 'suspect' and as in a good detective story, it is possible to be misled by 'false' clues into a blind alley. Sometimes there are simply not enough clues or information to make a perfect 'deduction'. Like a detective who may resort to fingerprints or DNA of hair or blood, a doctor also may only find the 'true suspect' by using sophisticated technology. Medicine, like crime detection, is an imperfect art, sometimes they get the wrong person! Doctors may use blood tests, X-rays, MRI or CAT scans, and also DNA tests. These are usually ordered to clarify what the doctor already suspects because of the particular collection of symptoms. They do not order tests if there is no indication, just as a detective does not interview or fingerprint people who were not suspects in the crime.'

It is possible to make this a fun process with a bright adolescent by asking them, if they were a doctor and a patient presented with a sore throat, a blocked nose, a fever, and aching limbs, what would they diagnose – a cold, glandular fever or flu? Discuss what extra evidence they might need to make a deduction (or diagnosis); what questions would a doctor ask the patient?

For example, length of time of symptoms; whether symptoms might include fatigue. Do they need a blood test for a cold? Why not?

Limiting factors for medical explanations

⊃ Parents who are over-confident in their own medical knowledge.
⊃ Parents who are anxiously preoccupied with medical information and who actually find focus on medical matters anxiety-provoking
⊃ Parents with limited language comprehension or cognitive capacity to understand the concepts.

Sometimes families of health professionals present for treatment. It is important that the treating therapist does not assume that medical terminology used in a familiar way is correctly understood.

It is important to guard against nominating additional symptoms that are characteristic of a condition but which are not currently present, as looking for signs of their appearance may lead the adolescent to increase what may also be hypervigilant behaviour.

Always check with the parent and adolescent the source of the information on their condition. They may already be alarmed by images of extreme versions of the condition viewed on TV, the internet or from neighbours' stories.

For parents or adolescents with limited ability to understand, presenting single pieces of information in simple forms supported by simple handouts can be helpful. Repetition of the simplified ideas on a regular basis is helpful.

Common questions

Parents may ask the following questions.

'Why doesn't the doctor order tests that I want?'

Therapist's answer: 'A good diagnostician only uses tests for which there is an indication, and where a test will prove or disprove their hypothesis. Patients are not trained to know these indications. Sometimes a doctor will order a test to put a patient's (or their own) mind at rest. Tests are expensive and doctors are discouraged from over-investigating.'

'What causes this problem? What is 'pathology'?'

Therapist's answer: 'Pathology is the naming of the underlying processes within the body that cause disease and dysfunction. Every disease has a unique collection of processes that characterise that disease. These may (or may not) result in symptoms. For instance, the pathology associated with cancer is abnormal growth of cells. Hence the creation of lumps or extra white cells in blood that cause leukaemia. This abnormal growth of cells causes different effects or symptoms. These symptoms are what the doctor or patient notice, and each condition presents different symptoms.'

'Sometimes in early phases of a disease there may be not symptoms but the underlying pathology is still there. A doctor can tell that the collection of symptoms that present as aching in the muscles and joints, accompanied by a headache and fever is not arthritis because (a) the joints are not swollen; (b) a headache and fever are present; (c) the pain and fever have occurred in the last few days rather than in the pattern that characterises arthritis. Without any additional information (e.g. recent travel to the tropics) the doctor is likely to deduce that the patient has the flu. If the patient has just returned from the tropics the doctor may need to consider rarer contagious diseases that exist only in the tropics.'

'What do I do when I get contradictory advice?'

Therapist's answer: 'It is helpful to have one treating doctor who is in charge of co-ordinating all referrals and the resultant opinions, advice and information. This may be a paediatrician or general practitioner or the most frequently seen specialist. One specialist may ask for a second opinion from another in the same field in order to confirm their opinion. It is possible for doctors to disagree but ultimately there is usually enough consensus for an agreed treatment path. Where conflicting opinions have occurred, this may mean seeking an independent third opinion. In hospitals where many different specialists have been involved or where there has been lack of clarity or multiple disagreements, a case conference may be suggested. A case conference is where all treating practitioners meet to put all the known evidence forward at one time and where different opinions are aired and discussion among everyone occurs until an agreed outcome is reached. Case conferences are rare because they are expensive, difficult to organise and usually occur as a last resort.'

'Should I keep looking until I get an answer?'

Therapist's answer: 'There are three problems with mounting a continuous search for certainty. Firstly, certainty may not happen; secondly, it may not change what you have to do; thirdly, searching delays all the actions necessary to resume a fulfilling life. At the end of the search these actions may be all that is possible and in the meantime, growing and learning time is lost.'

'There is yet another consequence of continually searching. As the study of pain is a specialty area itself, not all doctors are aware of the most recent developments. Doctors are trained to find an answer and usually want to help and so will always keep searching in their particular area of specialty. They may produce more and more remote and rare explanations, which becomes more and more confusing. This is what produces the 'fat file' of the chronic pain patient.' [Described in Chapter 1.]

'It can seem that only when you have certainty can you know what to do, or that there may be something as yet undiscovered. Not having a name for the pain or a diagnosis may seem unsatisfactory. However, we know from relatively recent research that there is underlying pathology in the nervous system itself to explain a lowered pain threshold causing greater sensitivity to pain. If all appropriate referrals have been made and tests have been completed, then it is reasonable to assume that what may seem a 'grey' area of pain neurophysiology may be the only explanation possible.'

Common tools of the detective/doctor's trade

Most tests that are used by doctors have clear simple explanations available on the internet. Sitting with the adolescent or parent and talking through the details can be appropriate and helpful. Misinformation can cause anxiety.

Common blood tests

There are many sophisticated blood tests a specialist or general practitioner doctor may require in order to make a diagnosis. Blood tests can measure:

⊃ hormone levels in the blood to diagnose deficiency or overproduction of endocrine glands

⊃ the presence of an inflammatory process in the body. Erythrocyte sedimentation rate (ESR) measures the stickiness of small cells (platelets) in the blood. It is an indirect measure of inflammation which can be caused by infections (viral or bacterial) or by non-infectious conditions (such as arthritis). A raised ESR is only one of a number of signs that indicate arthritis. It is possible to have a raised ESR from other causes.

X-rays

An X-ray takes a picture of the body's skeleton and other organs such as lungs, etc., where there is a suspicion of disease. As X-ray is unable to pass through dense structures so bones appear as white images against the black background. Other dense matter such as lumps, cysts, cancers, foreign bodies, fractures and dislocations are similarly revealed. X-rays may also reveal abnormal density including a deficiency in calcium in bones.

Bone-density test

This test is ordered where poor bone density is suspected, e.g. following longstanding inactivity. Densiometry gives a rating that compares to a normal range, and it is more conclusive than an X-ray.

Soft tissues which are not revealed by X-rays can be revealed by the following tests, each of which reveals different degrees of detail. In general they are listed in order from the least expensive to the most costly.

Ultrasound

Ultrasound is based on sound waves emitted by a probe. The wave is turned back by solid tissues in the body and appears on a screen so that when beamed on a torn tendon, for instance, it will reveal the break in the tendon.

CAT scans

Computerised axial tomography (CAT) scans take radiographic pictures of slices through the body from different angles, which, when put together, give a three-dimensional appearance. (Rather like slices of a lemon that would reveal the details of the inside of the lemon, which, when put together, constructs the whole. This would show where the pips were; how deep they were, and the pattern of the internal membranes.) CAT scans reveal abnormalities of blood vessels, muscle tendons, as well as lumps, cysts and foreign bodies. CAT scans reveal more detail than an ultrasound and are capable of greater penetration, deeper into the body.

MRI

Magnetic resonant imaging (MRI) is a further development of a CAT scan, revealing even more detail but at much greater cost to the public or private purse. Where no evidence of damage is shown in a CAT scan, an MRI may still find evidence of damage such as a very fine stress fracture.

Nerve conduction tests

These are used to determine whether there is a block or delay in conductivity of the passage of an impulse down a nerve. The most common use is where there is compression in the median nerve at the site of the wrist as the nerve passes through a fibrous tunnel.

The medical specialist

Some specialty areas overlap.

Anaesthetists' area of expertise is the study of anaesthesia, or the body's nervous systems responsible for awareness of sensations, including pain. Anaesthetists use drugs to put patients to sleep so that no sensation is experienced during operations. They also use drugs to manage pain following operations.

Orthopaedic surgeons are doctors whose area of specialty is the skeleto-muscular system. They study and operate on the structure and function of bones and joints.

Neurologists' specialty is the study of the nervous system. Neurologists are often the first doctor a family will see for headaches to exclude lesions or damage to nerves in the brain. They will test the function of nerves following injury.

Rheumatologists specialise in conditions that involve systemic diseases of the body that produce changes in joints or muscles, such as juvenile arthritis, psoriasis, fibromyalgia or complex regional pain syndrome.

Gastroenterologists study the gastro-intestinal tract which includes the ingestion and digestion of food, including the elimination of waste products in the faeces.

Gynaecologists have specialist knowledge of the female reproductive organs and processes including menstruation and pregnancy.

Endocrinologists study the endocrine glands which control complex systems in the body that are responsible for fertility, growth and metabolism. For instance, a dysfunction of the thyroid gland due to iodine deficiency can cause abnormal decrease or increase in metabolism. Malfunction of the ovaries can cause menstrual pain.

Urologists study the renal system. This includes the structure and function of the urinary tract, bladder, kidneys and all the tubes that convey urine.

Paediatricians study the medical conditions pertaining to children and adolescents.

Ophthalmologists study diseases of the eyes.

Conditions associated with chronic pain

There are many other medical conditions in which chronic pain occurs. Some examples are neurofibromatosis, sickle-cell anaemia, interstitial cystitis and post-operative complications such as nerve entrapment, tethering or scarring. There are many others. The conditions chosen to elaborate on here have been selected because they are more common and likely to be treated in community settings rather than in specialist medical clinics in large hospitals. However, should a therapist be required to assist in the management of the chronic pain associated with the more rare conditions, most aspects of this book are relevant.

Neuropathic pain

Neuropathic pain is pain arising from abnormalities in the pain-transmission system. This may be caused by trauma (including limb amputation and post-operative nerve entrapment) or disease of nervous tissue (e.g. polyneuropathy from diabetes). Complex regional pain syndrome Type I (CRPS I) (sometimes known as reflex sympathetic dystrophy) also produces neuropathic pain. Experiences of abnormal sensation (dysaesthesia), or heightened pain sensation from a normal stimulus such as touch (allodynia), or lowered pain threshold and increased sensitivity to pain (hyperalgesia) can result. Pain can be burning, throbbing or feel like needles or an electric shock; it may be spontaneous and disproportionate to objective findings. When symptoms are typical of neuropathic pain and other causative factors are excluded, patients should be treated as having a pain-transmission syndrome.[2]

Recurrent headaches

There is a detailed classification of headaches developed by the International Headache Society. The most common types of recurrent headaches in children and adolescents are migraine and tension-type headache (TTH). There is considerable discrepancy between parent and adolescent, and between teacher and adolescent reporting of headache. It is therefore important to evaluate the frequency and intensity of the headache from the adolescent's report. Headaches are the most frequently reported somatic complaint in schoolchildren and adolescents and the most frequently investigated pain complaint in this non-clinical population. In addition, headache complaints are more likely to be accompanied by other pain complaints. Estimates of migrainous headache prevalence rates vary from 3% to 11% with most sufferers experiencing attacks less than once a month and 30% estimated to experience more frequent attacks. Girls have a higher incidence of both types of headache. The prevalence of attacks increases with the age of the adolescent. The prognosis for improvement without intervention is poor, with the prognosis being less positive for girls.[3]

Pathophysiology of headaches

Migraine has been thought to be due to vascular and neurogenic changes. Biochemical mechanisms may cause vasoconstriction followed by vasodilatation and inflammation, with pain arising from the pial arteries and the sensitisation of nociceptors around the arteries. Migraines have been found to be 50% genetically determined in adults, with the genetic factor being stronger in females.

Tension-type headache (TTH) has been thought to arise from increased tension in muscles as a learned response to stress. School children with frequent TTH have been shown to have increased sensitivity to pressure stimuli in pericranial muscles and lowered pain thresholds, possibly due to the longstanding pain disorder.

Other contributing factors

Irregular, poor or extended sleep over weekends and irregular meals have been found to elicit migraine attacks in children. There is only a small subgroup of migraine sufferers who appear to have sensitivity to foods.

Mental and physical stress is more often a trigger in TTH. These adolescents are not exposed to higher levels of external stressors but their perception of stress is more negative with feelings of pressure and frustration, fear of failure, problems with others and bullying identified. Headaches arise frequently during school hours but most children with TTH headache do not miss school and function well in spite of pain. School absenteeism is more frequent in children with migraines, with the intensity of the headache relating to the degree of disability. Children who seek help for headaches are likely to have severe or unusual headaches, including a combination of migraine and TTH. It is suggested that school attendance or medication use is not a reliable measure of treatment outcome, but that social functioning such as peer relations, leisure and school work may be better measures.

Headaches may result from trauma such as a head injury.

Treatments

Cognitive behavioural therapy (CBT) and relaxation training on a one-to-one basis have been found to be effective in reducing frequency and intensity of TTH and non-organic migraine (*see* Chapter 7). School-based programmes with a trained therapist are also effective. Home-based programmes are less effective with adolescents who monitor their headaches showing no improvement. Pharmacological treatments are available. Medications need to be prescribed by a paediatrician, neurologist or general practitioner, with recommendations to take the medication at the first sign of the headache.

Recurrent abdominal pain

Recurrent abdominal pain (RAP) occurs predominantly in girls in middle childhood aged 7–11 years. Adolescents presenting with a different chronic pain condition may describe experiences of RAP in earlier school years. RAP was first identified in 1958 following a study of 1000 school children in Bristol.[4] The study concluded that RAP rarely had an identifiable organic basis and occurred in 10% of the population; that emotional disturbance is more common in children with RAP which is frequently associated with other somatic symptoms. Also, that other family members had a higher incidence of somatic complaints and abdominal pain. Later studies raised the possibility that the distress associated with RAP may be a consequence rather than a cause of the pain since children with organically based pain recorded similar levels of distress.[5] It is suggested that adolescents with pain-related disability may have had their behaviour and environment shaped by the earlier experience of RAP with parents and peers responding to the established sick role. Parent's caretaking role may increase their child's dependency, with the child not acquiring the adaptive skills such as ability to endure discomfort or seek peer-related support. All of these factors would impact on any pain experienced in adolescents when independent managing would normally occur.[6]

Musculo-skeletal pain

Musculo-skeletal pain can include diffuse pain from hypermobility; fibromyalgia; arthritis; or more localised pain in a limb (including complex regional pain syndrome), neck, knee or back. It may result in over-use syndromes. Girls appear to have more persistent pain than boys with the risk for persistent pain increasing 1.2 times per year of age with neck pain the most persistent. Early studies suggest that between 15% and 27% of schoolchildren have significant limb pain.[7]

Complex regional pain syndrome (CRPS)

This condition, which has also been called reflex sympathetic dystrophy, has been classified since 1994 by the International Association for the Study of Pain (IASP), as CRPS type I or CRPS type II (Causalgia). CRPS I, often initiated following a minor injury, is characterised by positive sensory abnormalities including spontaneous pain or pain on movement which is out of keeping with the original injury; vascular abnormalities including colour and temperature changes; oedema, including swelling or sweating and motor/trophic changes such as weakness and tremor; nail or hair changes; co-ordination deficits, or joint stiffness. Diagnosis is made if three of these changes are evident with two or more signs from each category present. Prolonged disuse of a limb may result in changes in bone density in the affected limb, measurable by a bone-density test. CRPS II exhibits similar signs and symptoms but a lesion of the peripheral nerve structures and subsequent focal deficits are mandatory for diagnosis, and in addition symptoms and signs spread beyond the innervation territory of the injured nerve.

Studies in the adult research literature show cortical changes such as increased synaptic efficiency that means less stimulus is required to activate pain mechanisms, and pain that fluctuates with sensory and non-sensory (psychosocial) inputs; imagined movement is sufficient to cause an increase in pain, with reduced distance between cortical representation of the affected area and adjacent areas, similar to findings in phantom limb pain (remapping). Adult CRPS I studies have demonstrated signs of neglect with human and animal studies suggesting that disuse of a limb can generate signs and symptoms of CRPS I. New theories propose a mismatch between motor commands and appropriate sensory feedback (possibly caused by cortical remapping), the conflict resulting in pain.[8] Differences in outcome and treatment exist between adult populations with CRPS I and adolescent populations, with outcomes for adolescents better than those for adult populations. The use of TENS machines is more effective in adolescents than in adults.[9]

What has been concluded by most specialists is that the earlier treatment is instituted, the better the outcome. Clinically, it is possible for an adolescent to present with insufficient signs to make a diagnosis of CRPS I, yet sufficient distress and dysfunction to still require management. For some adolescents, a neural block may assist in allowing a pain-free period in which a movement programme may begin. The main goals of therapy are pain relief and restoration of function with a graduated programme of mobilisation and desensitisation. A multidisciplinary approach which includes physiotherapy, occupational therapy, psychological counselling and anaesthiology has been found to be the most successful.

Juvenile primary fibromyalgia syndrome (JPFS)

JPFS is found in children as young as five years of age and is characterised by widespread chronic pain accompanied by fatigue, poor sleep and other non-musculoskeletal symptoms such as irritable bowel syndrome. JPFS is most commonly diagnosed in adolescent girls aged between 13 and 15 years with significant psychosocial impact on the adolescent and family, including school absences due to pain. While most studies describe adult fibromyalgia (earlier called fibrositis), differences between adults and adolescents have been noted.

It is suggested that for diagnosis, adolescents must have pain in only three sites for a period greater than three months, in addition to five or more activated tender points and must meet three of ten minor criteria – such as anxiety, poor sleep, IBS, fatigue, or headaches.[10]

Researchers have noted the overlap between fibromyalgia and chronic fatigue syndrome. Some researchers have proposed that joint hypermobility may be a contributing factor. Familial aggregation occurs, with one study finding evidence of a contributing gene, another finding the 71% of children with fibromyalgia have mothers with fibromyalgia. Other factors suggested in the literature are sedentary lifestyle impacting on quality of sleep, emotional distress (as this is common to other pain conditions it is unlikely to be causal in nature) and neurohormonal changes affecting sleep.

A meta-analysis of the adult literature showed that low doses of antidepressants led to some improvements; however, cognitive behaviour therapy and exercise alone or in combination with pharmacologic treatment showed larger effect sizes than pharmacological therapy alone.[11] A more recent study has found evidence for improved function in adolescents treated with a cognitive behavioural programme.[12] However, unstandardised diagnostic criteria remain a problem in research with some doctors questioning the validity of the diagnosis as a physical disorder.

Hypermobility

Joint hypermobility describes an increased range of joint or spinal movement found in 10–30% of the population. It is more common in females than in males, and more common in people of Asian and African origin than in Caucasians. Benign joint hypermobility should be distinguished from joint hypermobility syndrome (JHS) with which it shares the common feature of lax joints and increased pain. JHS is defined by the Brighton 1998 classification. It is familial and is distinguished by chronic musculoskeletal pain, fatigue, soft tissue and visceral injury, skin abnormalities and neurogenic dysfunction. Subgroups of JHS include Ehlers-Danlos syndrome, Marfan's syndrome and ontogenesis imperfecta.

Arthritis

Juvenile rheumatoid arthritis (JRA) is a diagnosis covering polyarticular JRA involving more than five joints, and pauciarticular JRA involving four or fewer joints. The disease is characterised by high intermittent fever and rash initially, and pain and swelling most commonly in the small joints of the hands, knees, elbows, ankles and feet. Studies have shown that there are lowered pain thresholds at areas of inflammation and in non-inflamed paraspinal areas. Lowered pain thresholds persist beyond times of active inflammation, suggesting central and peripheral sensitisation. Some evidence exists that levels of pain do not necessarily correlate with disease severity. Treatment usually involves pharmacological intervention and while 'prospective or experimental studies have not yet confirmed that psychosocial factors directly influence pain in JRA', some psychological treatments in the form of cognitive behavioural treatments such as relaxation, biofeedback and meditation may help.[13]

Back pain

Back pain is common in children and adolescents and increases with age, with the steepest increase occurring between 13 and 14 years. Usually there is no trauma or pathology to explain the pain. It appears that only children experiencing more severe pain seek help. Various risk factors have been explored, including anthropometric differences, decreased flexibility of hamstrings and trunk and back muscle strength. Although differences in physical measures have been found, it is unknown whether these are causal or secondary to the pain. Suggested treatments are not empirically validated but follow guidelines for adult back pain. These include discouragement of extended resting and resumption of normal activities.

Knee pain

Knee pain is relatively common in adolescents with some studies reporting a 29–32% prevalence with possible causes other than trauma, sited as joint laxity, patellar instability, congenital synovial plica, hamstring tightness and structural abnormalities of the foot. Knee pain is more prevalent in adolescents who have been active in regular sport. It is usually worse after activity, and a proportion of these adolescents are required to stop playing sport. A chondromalacia patella is diagnosed when changes to the cartilage of the knee caps (patellae) occur.

Osgood-Schlatters is a disease that also causes pain and swelling in the knee at the top of the shin bone where the patellar tendons connect the muscles to the knee. It is unlikely to become chronic pain if relieved by appropriate rest.

Symptoms secondary to persistent pain

Many adolescents develop secondary symptoms as a result of longstanding pain. These can become almost a condition on their own. A vicious cycle of pain and inactivity lead to deconditioning with continuous feelings of fatigue being a daily barrier to resumption of activity on top of the pain. (*See* Chapter 10.) Similarly, pain that affects sleep adds to this vicious cycle of fatigue and leads to significant sleep disorders. (*See* Chapter 4.)

References

1 Jensen MP, Nielson WR, Romano JM, *et al*. Patient beliefs predict patient functioning: further support for a cognitive-behavioural model of chronic pain. *Pain*. 1999; **81**: 95–104.

2 Olsson GL. Neuropathic pain in children. In: McGrath PJ, Finley DA, editors. *Chronic and Recurrent Pain in Children and Adolescents*. Seattle: IASP Press; 1999, pp. 85–98.

3 Larsson B. Recurrent headaches in children and adolescents. In: McGrath PJ, Finley DA, editors. *Chronic and Recurrent Pain in Children and Adolescents.* Seattle: IASP Press; 1999, pp. 115–40.

4 Apley J, Naish N. Recurrent abdominal pain: a field survey of 1,000 children with recurrent abdominal pain. *Arch Dis Child.* 1958; **33**: 165–70.

5 Walker LS, Greene JW. Children with recurrent abdominal pain and their parents: more somatic complaints, anxiety, and depression than other patient families? *J Ped Psychol.* 1989; **14**: 231–4.

6 Walker LS. The evolution of research on recurrent abdominal pain: history, assumptions, and a conceptual model. In: McGrath PJ, Finley DA, editors. *Chronic and Recurrent Pain in Children and Adolescents.* Seattle: IASP Press; 1999, pp. 141–73.

7 McGrath PJ, Breau L. Musculoskeletal pain. In: McGrath PJ, Finley DA, editors. *Chronic and Recurrent Pain in Children and Adolescents.* Seattle: IASP Press; 1999, pp. 173–97.

8 McCabe CS, Haigh RC, Halligan PW, *et al.* Simulating sensory-motor incongruence in healthy volunteers: implications for a cortical model of pain. *Rheum.* 2005; **44**: 509–16.

9 Taylor LM. Complex regional pain syndrome: comparing adults and adolescents. *Topics in Advanced Practice Nursing eJournal.* 2002; **2**(2). © Medscape Portals Inc.

10 Yunis MB, Masi AT. Juvenile primary fibromyalgia syndrome: a clinical study of thirty-three patients and matched normal controls. *Arthritis Rheum.* 1985; **28**: 138–45.

11 Kashikar-Zuck S, Graham TB, Huenefeld MD, Powers SW. A review of bio-behavioural research in juvenile primary fibromyalgia syndrome. *Arthritis Care and Research.* 2000; **13**(6): 388–97.

12 Kashikar-Zuck S, Swain NF, Jones BA, *et al.* Efficacy of cognitive-behavioural intervention for juvenile primary fibromyalgia syndrome. *J Rheum.* 2005; **32**(8): 1594–602.

13 McGrath PJ, Breau L. Musculoskeletal pain. In: McGrath PJ, Finley DA, editors. *Chronic and Recurrent Pain in Children and Adolescents.* Seattle: IASP Press; 1999, p. 177.

CHAPTER 3

Pain and the family

HOW FAMILIES CONTRIBUTE

CHAPTER SUMMARY

This chapter examines the effect of pain on the family and the influence of family culture on the adolescent and their pain. There is a brief examination of the place of the developing adolescent within the family, and the issues that arise for the individual adolescent are outlined. Assessment of behaviours and parenting style form the background to some suggestions on how to assist in the management of unhelpful practices such as: the stalemate caused by waiting for an answer; unhelpful family stories, and behaviours around pain flare-ups. Positive suggestions for replacement behaviours and encouraging independence are made. Other family problems that influence the outcome for the adolescent are identified with case studies to illustrate.

Background

Restrictions on daily life are not confined only to the adolescent experiencing the difficulty. Families living with a child with pain report distress.[1] Family activities may be restricted, a parent may stop work to stay at home, siblings may feel neglected, and parents may sleep in separate rooms, all in order to cope with the adolescent dealing with persistent pain.[2] Parenting styles, parent–child relationships, family conflict and family 'culture' affect how an adolescent manages pain – 'illness episodes are important socialising events for children'.[3,4,5] Parent responses contribute to the sick-role behaviour.[6] Some families and cultures externalise and verbalise suffering, other families are stoic and internalising.[7] Differences in symptom reporting can be due to cultural variations in child rearing practices, as can parental socio-economic status and values.[8] The early literature in social learning theory is predominantly in the adult pain population.[9,10,11,12] However, there is some literature specific to the paediatric and adolescent population.[13]

Mothers have been described as having a 'gatekeeper' role in the family when, in stressed families, they take on the role of protecting the children from further psychological distress. Fathers' involvement is a protective factor against psychological maladjustment in adolescents from separated families, and psychological distress in women.[14] However, fathers frequently feel excluded.[15] It is mothers who appear to be the most significant in the parent–child relationship around pain. One study showed situations in which children report greater depressive and anxiety symptoms and those children, who reported their mother as solicitous in various pain situations, had greater child-reported functional disability.[16] Adolescents who did not cope well with chronic pain had mothers who were more involved with their children's participation in an exercise task and exhibited behaviour that discouraged the adolescent's efforts to cope with the task.[17] Other studies showed that: adolescents experience the most rewarding by parents in pain situations and more rewarding by peers in a pain-free situation.[18] This outcome is an obvious reason for the adolescent with pain to attend school!

Adolescents with recurrent unexplained pain and their parents were more likely to report some positive consequences of pain (e.g. getting extra time in exams or having fun while staying at home), and to identify models of pain or illness in their environment than were children with explained pain.[19] This is a powerful argument for education and an explanation of diagnosis and pain as described in Chapters 1 and 2.

Children learn behaviour through observation of and interaction with a parent with chronic low back pain.[20]

Parent/child relationship problems, particularly in the mother and child, were associated with avoidant coping and internalising of emotions while avoidant coping in turn is associated with poor coping with persistent pain.[21,22] (*See* Chapter 6.)

Parents of adolescents who reported high levels of disability, depression and anxiety had parents who also had clinically significant levels of depression, anxiety and parental stress. The greatest levels of adolescent depression were shown by the youngest adolescents who had the greatest chronicity of the problem.[23]

Studies have shown that relative differences and relationships in the families of adolescents with persistent pain, fall *within the context of generally normative levels of parental and family functioning*. However, families of adolescents with persistent pain are characterised by unusual closeness (enmeshment) or lack of recognition of what is developmentally appropriate for the age of the adolescent. Conversely, families with psychologically healthy parents and families that are not characterised by high levels of enmeshment or conflict may be more likely to function adaptively with recurrent pain.[24]

The adolescent in the family

Families come in all forms – different-sex parents, same-sex parents, two generations or grandparents as parents, solo or separated parents, multiple siblings or no siblings. The adolescent exists within the unique environment of their family, placed as eldest, youngest, middle, etc. Families are often aware of their unique character, having agreed family stories to support this. They will describe themselves as 'rowdy', 'very close and loving', or alternatively, one girl described her family as a 'suck it up' family (i.e. a family where individuals accept and cope without support or communication with each other). Other families see themselves as victims of fate, collectively disabled, 'unlucky' and struggling against multiple health difficulties; X has a bad back, Y has migraines, Z has foot problems. (These may not be families with extreme physical disabilities such as those with congenital or hereditary problems.) Families with multiple family members with pain may not see the common theme of pain in their family. A number of studies show the prevalence of pain in families of adult chronic pain patients is significantly higher than in the general population.[25] Parents can serve as models for pain behaviour. Additionally, families differ in the ways in which they communicate feelings or emotions. For some, verbal expressions, discussions or enquiries about feelings are absent and the family operates only on a pragmatic, action-oriented level. Family members may not have an awareness of emotions or words for their feelings, whereas for others, the expression of feeling states is heightened and observable as pain behaviour, often expressed in catastrophic language.

The individual adolescent

In addition to the family, an adolescent faces many issues that may have been avoided, or lain dormant or unnoticed in their development in earlier childhood. In general these issues centre around their developing sexuality, independence and ability to cope. Self-assessment of abilities measured against those of peers, social acceptance in peer groups, self-esteem, individuation and emotional separation from parents are also issues. There is social pressure for achievement of independence and adulthood within the few short years of adolescence.

Adolescents with pain lasting more than three months (but of no documented physiological aetiology) show poor self-esteem, vague body symptoms and fears, difficulty in social contacts, fear of failure and not feeling socially accepted compared with a matched non-pain group.[26] The surfacing of these issues may explain why pain increases in the adolescent population.

Culture

Culture is defined as 'the way of life of a people. It consists of conventional patterns of thought and behaviour, including values, beliefs, rules of conduct, political organisation, economic activity, and the like, which are passed on from one generation to the next by learning – and not by inheritance.'[27] Culture would be expected to influence pain experience and behaviour beginning in early childhood. In addition, patterns of parent and other adult interactions with children in pain would be expected to reflect culturally based attitudes toward child-rearing, pain, and illness. These attitudes might also affect healthcare-seeking behaviour, decision and interactions with providers. An example of this may be where a family within an indigenous minority group fails to seek assistance from the dominant healthcare system because there are no indigenous healthcare workers and the family has had negative experiences with the dominant culture's authority structures.

A substantial number of studies demonstrate cultural differences in pain experience in specific settings (usually with adult populations). It is important not to stereotype, as many studies reflect that 'substantial *intracultural variation* exists within any cultural group'. It is recommended that practitioners reflect on culture and pain issues in local contexts.[28]

Parenting an adolescent with persistent pain

Relative differences and relationships in the families of adolescents with persistent pain *fall within the context of generally normative levels of parental and family functioning.* The subjective experience of being a parent of a child with persistent pain needs to be acknowledged by therapists. Parenting naturally requires a great deal of care and attention in the raising of a child. With rare exceptions, most parents have spent years striving to keep their child safe, to prevent, or relieve the pain and discomforts associated with the life of a child, i.e. hunger, cold, falls and accidents, unsafe environments, unfair teachers or peers, etc. It is usual practice for parents to advocate on behalf of their child at times of adversity. It is unrealistic – and indeed unkind – to expect that parents would not continue to demonstrate these qualities when they present for treatment. It is a common experience of parents that they feel blamed when they are perceived as 'over' protective or over-involved in their attempts to relieve the pain; angry at the diagnostic vacuum, or pushy when advocating for resources or for fighting for 'proof' of the pain, on behalf of their child. They experience self-doubt and distress when they are unable to gain control over the pain and the repeated failures of treatment. Parents themselves may experience depression associated with their failure to change their child's pain.

It is the therapist's role to understand their subjective experience and to normalise their feelings without blame. This can be done in a number of ways that acknowledge the path the family has taken so far to get treatment. Any from the following list may apply to the parent's experience. Acknowledge: the burden of having an increasingly dependent child; the emotional distress of seeing their child in pain; the limitations of social and family functioning, including possible marital tensions between parents as to the management of the pain; the financial losses or career stresses that medical appointments have caused, plus the worry about the future development of the child.[29]

Assessment

It is important to assess the impact of the adolescent's chronic pain on the family and on the marital relationship in order to understand the family's subjective experience and the subsequent mental health problems that may exist, e.g. depression, anxiety, etc. It is also important to assess learning within the family environment that has predisposed the adolescent and their family to their current situation. An assessment of predisposing, precipitating and maintaining factors in a case formulation is a helpful place from which to start. A developmental history by a psychologist is likely to provide valuable information. This would include an assessment of attachment styles, parenting style and inter-relational patterns within the family. The biopsychosocial formulation grid in Chapter 1 takes social learning and psychological development into account and may help the therapist in understanding the adolescent and family. A detailed understanding of behaviours that occur with pain flare-up is necessary to comprehend family engagement with pain and pain behaviours.

Issues to be addressed with parents

Evidence in the research literature as well as clinical observation underpins these recommendations.

Unexplained pain

Address the unexplained nature of any pain with clarification of diagnosis and pain physiology education that includes information about modelling, social learning and the influence of thoughts and feelings on pain (*see* Chapters 1 and 2). It can be more acceptable if presented indirectly as general knowledge, using examples not necessarily based around pain. Having time between sessions to digest the impact of this information can also help the family with the process of acceptance. For some, however, this information becomes immediately personal and is too challenging. They perceived the information as a form of blaming of themselves for their child's pain. Or it may be that the prospect of what lies ahead is simply too uncomfortable to contemplate. (*See* 'yellow flags' in Chapter 5.)

Waiting for an answer

Discuss the consequences of 'waiting for an answer' if all investigations have revealed nothing. Give an example of how it feels to be waiting for a phone call. In this situation you are in limbo, you can only do fill-in activities. You can't make big decisions that will get your day moving; you don't want to start anything that takes you away from the main game, i.e. listening for the phone. If you started something you might suddenly have to change directions because of the phone call. In this instance it can help to propose an hypothesis for the likely cause of the pain, and then to plan actions that you and the adolescent and family would do if that hypothesis were true. If progress is made, then one can assume this could be the right track.

Pain flare-up

Assess what happens when a pain flare-up occurs by asking for a detailed account of the last time pain flared up. (This is useful information to know about other family members' pain behaviours as well.)

Where did the flare-up occur? Who was there? What was everybody doing? How did they know there was pain? What did their child do or say? Did it occur suddenly or gradually? What had happened just prior to the increase in pain? What was said and what action was taken? Was there any action taken by the adolescents themselves to manage the pain?

Family stories

Ask how the parent sees their child. 'They are just like me – a real worrier.' Are there family stories around the family or individuals? (There are often formative events around which these stories are constructed.) Parents may describe one child as 'sensitive' or 'good', or another as coping less, or as more 'resilient'. 'I remember how he didn't like his teacher in grade one and he refused to go to school', or 'I am very lucky – she's so good, a real companion.'

Remind the parent that their child gets a large part of their sense of themself from people in their environment reflecting back to them what they are like. If events or stories are repeated, they will eventually think, 'I must be like that!' As parents they have the greatest influence over their child even though it might not feel like that at times. And for this reason it is helpful to choose stories about their child that describe coping attributes, e.g. 'He hated his grade one teacher but he made himself go to school despite that, he has often been able to get over his difficulties like this' – help them find other examples.

Managing independently

Ask the adolescent and parent if there is *anything* that any other person can do that takes the pain away. Give time for this discussion, as acceptance of this is fundamental to acceptance of recommendations that can seem challenging. (Not attending to pain behaviours, etc.) If it is agreed that no other person relieves or removes the pain, it may be possible to get an agreement with parent and adolescent for new independent managing. Stress that independence does not mean leaving the adolescent isolated and unsupported. This strategy is to allow space for the adolescents first and foremost to have the experience of managing for themselves. Remind them of the effect of belief in ability to manage pain on pain itself, by reiterating Bandura's study on self-efficacy as set out in Chapter 1.[30]

A useful analogy in discussion with parents can be to ask if they remember what they did in teaching their child to dress independently – they modelled the dressing behaviour daily themselves; they indicated that they expected that the child would try to do it; they gave them the opportunity, i.e. they made clothes available and stepped back to let them attempt the dressing. Then they encouraged any attempt, however imperfect. Eventually, the child assumed full responsibility without argument because dressing became a skill. In the same way, pain management can also be a skill.

> *Parents need to feel the therapist's compassion and concern for the well-being of their child.*

Assure the parent that their child will work out and practise strategies for managing their pain flare-up with the support of the therapist. (*See* Chapters 6 and 7.) Parents often find this challenging and find it difficult to 'let go' of this aspect of the protective role they have performed in the early years in their child's life. Listening to any feelings of uncertainty, loss or anxiety from the parent (usually the mother, but possibly supported by father) is important.

Replacement behaviours

Suggest new, replacement behaviours by the parent that will support their child's new behaviours, modifying them to make it workable for the family (*see* Handout 4: Managing pain behaviours). It can be helpful to have a family meeting with siblings to discuss these changes and what they can do as well. It is important to go through each point with the parent and to discuss how this will work for them at home and how they will manage. It is very important to listen to parents' concerns and to modify the suggestions as required. This may entail changing the handout by making shorter points or doing only some of the changed behaviours suggested, thereby testing out the family's tolerances.

Lifestyle regulation

Help the parent and adolescent regulate their environment and personal lifestyle habits. In the area of managing persistent pain, longstanding habits involving poor sleep routines require regulating (*see* Chapter 4).[31] An adolescent with persistent headaches needs food and fluid intake regulated. Helping a parent in this process may entail the therapist equipping the adolescent with skills for managing the required behaviour, e.g. relaxation or a pre-bed plan (*see* Chapters 4 and 7), listening to the needs of each party and negotiating a contract to which both parties agree.

Trial and follow up the new behaviours giving attention to:
- *any* positive change (don't let the words 'I tried' inadvertently imply inability or failure – remind them that even initiating a new action is progress)
- the parent's experience and feelings around the new behaviour. If the new behaviours cause distress or worry, these feelings must be addressed with counselling support for the parent.

Common statements from parents who are challenged by their child's new independence are:
- 'I worry that my child won't tell me when there is something wrong'
- 'I believe my child will . . . repress their feelings . . . feel isolated, alone in their pain'
- 'I will lose the close relationship that we have where he/she tells me everything'
- 'They will feel I am not there for them'.

(*See* '🔑 yellow flags' in this chapter.)

Pain in family members

Assist the family in finding assistance for other family members who have chronic pain. It is not helpful as a therapist to attempt to assist your adolescent's parent who has chronic pain. Find alternative sources of assistance and, if possible, with the adolescent's and parent's permission, discuss with their therapist ways in which the adult's pain and pain behaviours can be managed so as to not involve the adolescent. This may require getting help from outside the home for chores.

It can be helpful in some parent–child relationships to have a discussion about appropriate communication around the parent's pain. Examples might be:
- 'Do not talk about your pain but, if necessary, ask for assistance only if it is needed rather than as a 'special favour''
- 'Do not expect the adolescent to do more than what might be a normal number of chores. Keep these within the bounds of their abilities'
- 'If pain is worse at any time and you feel your mood or manner is likely

to be affected, simply mention that it is a bad day today but you know
how to manage it yourself'
- ⊃ 'Do not allow any observable pain behaviours such as groaning, clutching
the painful place etc.'

Marital disharmony

Sometimes in the process of looking at family issues for an adolescent, marital
tensions become evident. This may be a significant stressor for the adolescent,
which impacts on pain.[32] Advising the parents to seek help and assisting in an
appropriate referral will be helpful for the adolescent as it will lessen anxiety
levels and allow them to concentrate only on managing their pain.

It is useful to have suggestions to manage pain behaviours for parents.
Having a written form can assist in shaping a discussion on each point and
how the parent will execute the recommendation. To some degree, having a
written handout also normalises the recommendations in that they present as
something that is 'normally' presented to parents, i.e. other parents have also
needed this guidance. It diminishes what is a very common feeling of guilt and
self-blame that parents experience, namely that they somehow 'got it wrong'
and are a failure as a parent.

The following is a handout to *use as a basis for discussion* with parents
(*see also* Handout 4 in the Appendix). Some aspects may be modified, e.g.
an agreed discussion time may be arranged if parent and child are distressed
about the 'no discussion' suggestion.

Managing pain behaviours

Pain behaviour is associated with increasing the areas in the brain that are
responsive to pain, thereby increasing sensitivity to pain. In other words,
decreasing pain behaviour decreases the experience of pain.

Positive reinforcement is a response to your child's behaviour that will
increase the likelihood of the behaviour occurring again. **Attention** for pain
behaviour is a very powerful reinforcer for children.
- ⊃ Emphasise that you are unable to take your child's pain away, but say
that she/he will receive lots of love and attention (not about pain or pain
behaviour) and given rewards for coping.
- ⊃ Ignore any pain behaviours exhibited by your child (verbal groaning,
crying, guarding).
- ⊃ Give special attention and praise for coping behaviours (relaxation and
breathing techniques have been taught, along with visualisation).
- ⊃ Do not enter into a discussion with your child regarding her pain and
function, e.g. walk away.

Do not . . .
- ⊃ assume responsibility for anything your child can do themself
- ⊃ use punishment or assess their progress negatively in front of your child

➲ focus on the illness behaviours or give attention for pain behaviour
➲ ask how she/he is feeling or how much pain she/he has
➲ give excessive reassurance
➲ focus attention on the symptoms or show concern (even though you may feel it!)
➲ attend to your child when she/he is in pain or in discomfort
➲ believe your child is vulnerable and unable to cope.

Do ...

➲ give attention during symptom-free periods (e.g. 'you are working well', and 'you are doing well')
➲ be aware of demands for positioning; they are probably requests for attention
➲ expect your child to function in spite of physical distress (this is not cruel but actually therapeutic as your child will be convinced of their ability to manage by the experience of success)
➲ be firm – this communicates the conviction that your child is strong enough and competent enough to overcome this distress
➲ believe that your child can increase her functioning
➲ treat your child as an active agent in her treatment
➲ help your child to problem solve about how to actively change things, e.g. 'what can you do about this?'
➲ reduce parental concern if the opportunity arises
➲ be aware of how you feel towards your child
➲ follow through with times and expectations put into place
➲ support all members of the treating team.

(*Courtesy of Sophia Franks*)

Parents need to be taught new skills to understand and negotiate this process of change. Helping the adolescent regulate their environment and personal habits requires the negotiating of boundaries and the placing of limits on extremes of behaviour. In the area of managing persistent pain, longstanding habits involving poor sleep routines require regulating. (*See* Chapter 4.) This is especially relevant for an adolescent with persistent headaches who needs regular food and fluid intake. Helping a parent in this process may entail the therapist equipping the adolescent with skills for managing the required behaviour, e.g. relaxation or a pre-bed plan (*see* Chapter 4), listening to the needs of each party and negotiating a contract to which both parties agree.

Case study: Angela

Angela was an adolescent who was diagnosed with complex regional pain syndrome (CRPS) in her leg. Despite having her CRPS managed, she continued to experience persistent leg pain, poor sleep and fatigue. She had difficulty getting to sleep and so talked to friends on her mobile phone or watched the TV in her room until 2.00 a.m. Her parents told her not to do this, but felt powerless in the face of their child's difficulties with pain and sleep. Her mother found her particularly difficult to wake in the morning and sometimes she missed school due to fatigue. Her grades at school were poor. In discussion with Angela, it appeared that she argued with her father in the family room so that he refused to let her to watch what she wanted. She blamed her father and the arguments for the habit she then developed of using the TV in her room as a way of getting to sleep.

Firstly sleep hygiene was discussed with Angela (*see* Chapter 10). She was taught relaxation strategies and she agreed that if she had difficulty getting to sleep, she would use these methods. She agreed to try this for three months. The therapist negotiated with the parents that particular programmes would be recorded on the family TV, or that Angela would be allowed to watch up until 10.30 p.m. Discussions with Angela and her father minimised conflict. No mobile phone conversations would be allowed after 9.30 p.m. And Angela, who was keen to learn to sleep, agreed to have her TV removed from her room.

At the end of the three months, Angela had learned to initiate sleep herself within an hour on most week nights. If she awoke she was able to get back to sleep easily using the same techniques. Her pain diminished as she became less tired and her school grades improved and she became more physically active. With her parents' help, she rewarded herself with a ticket to a special concert.

o━ 'Yellow flags'

Some parents relinquish parental responsibilities. They may describe their relationship with their child as that of 'best friends' or even as 'sisters'. This characteristic relationship may be evident when either party – but mostly the mother – frequently substitutes 'we' in places where the individual pronoun 'she' or 'I' is appropriate. Other noticeable characteristics may be colluding with, being amused by, or defending their child's inappropriate or unhelpful behaviours, i.e. generally abrogating parental responsibilities. This relationship may be a result of the individual parent's personality and psychopathology, or may develop, for example, in the case of an unsupported solo-parenting mother as result of the absence of an adult partner or perhaps with an absence of intimacy with an existing partner, such as an absent, workaholic father. For any child or adolescent, there is security in knowing that a parent is willing to act as an adult and take responsibility for setting limits, especially in issues of safety and well-being, and for making major decisions.

A child in pain can produce a change in the way parents relate. One parent may become over-involved to the exclusion of their partner; this is especially so if the parent (usually the mother) is taking responsibility for assisting their child in the night. It is a common occurrence that a child in pain ends up in the parental bed with the displaced parent in the child's bed. Alternatively, parents otherwise estranged can start to function together for the sake of their child. This is a factor in maintaining dysfunction for the adolescent. From their perspective (albeit unconscious), if the adolescent improves, the parents will resume their estrangement or even separate. An adolescent who remains unwell keeps the parents together.

Case study: Anthony

Anthony was a 14-year-old boy previously hospitalised for treatment and rehabilitation for symptoms associated with the complex regional pain syndrome (CRPS) of his left foot. The parents believed that his sacrum was 'malpositioned' and had spent a great deal of money on naturopathic medicines, manipulation and osteopathic treatments, in unsuccessful treatment for his CRPS. Anthony had a history of events involving headaches, weakness and fatigue labelled as 'chronic fatigue' by his parents. These events were associated with starting at secondary school, and a bullying event. At presentation in the pain management clinic, he was non-weight bearing and had extreme allodynia, needing a cradle in his bed to stop bedclothes touching his foot. He slept poorly. His mother was very attentive during his in-patient stay. His father, who had apparently always been uncommunicative, came infrequently. Over time it was apparent his parents had been experiencing marital discord for 18 months prior to Anthony's condition. His father had left the marital home for one year. Marital counselling had been attempted and treatment had been suggested for Anthony's father's depression. He had declined all attempts at help.

During the five months of naturopathic medicines and osteopathic treatments, and the increasing symptomatology of his CRPS, his father had moved back into the family home. He and Anthony's mother took turns to stay at home with Anthony who spent up to five hours at a time on his computer or on the couch. He had not attended school for 18 months.

A programme of intense physiotherapy, occupational therapy and psychological counselling, including pain education and pain-management strategies, returned full function to Anthony and a return to school was successful. During his counselling sessions, Anthony talked about his longstanding image of himself as a sick person who had little control over his body. He also spoke of how he habitually 'ran away' when he was frightened. He was unsure how he would handle his parents' impending separation on his return home. He was especially sensitive to his father's depression and passivity and felt very protective of him. Relapse strategies were discussed with him and ongoing local counselling was arranged.

On his return home, his parents separated again. Anthony continued to see his father independently but infrequently, describing the visits as 'difficult'.

On follow-up in six months' time, Anthony had once again stopped attending school, having been diagnosed as having chronic fatigue. He was once again homebound with his father staying several times a week to look after Anthony.

Comment

The causes of chronic fatigue syndrome are unknown at this time and while it is not presumed that this condition has its aetiology in Anthony's social and psychological situation, it is inescapable that his relapse caused a reinstatement of his preferred family situation, i.e. frequent (and more easily managed) contact with his father in the family home. At the same time, this new 'sickness', chronic fatigue syndrome, was consistent with what Anthony had acknowledged had been a belief established in early childhood about himself as a sick person. Anthony had chosen not to pursue his referral for ongoing psychotherapy, just as his father had not pursued treatment.

Parents differ in their awareness of their children's feelings and emotions. A family culture of high activity with no playtime or quiet recreation can be overwhelming (often for the youngest who has difficulty keeping up). There may be no space for a member of such a family to express their different need. Parents may spend time talking to their child about feelings rather than only about what they did in their day, e.g. 'How did you feel when X happened . . .?'

Families with a history of trauma or loss may not speak of these events within the family, the impact of the events remaining unacknowledged. Silence and secrecy impact on family function and are a dysfunctional means of coping. Examples may be: following the loss of a child, the remaining child may become 'precious' and overprotected; or painful relationships involving loss, such as the loss of a divorced or deceased partner, are not spoken of – leading to mystery around a person of significance in the adolescent's life.

A history of mental illness, a common one being post-natal depression in the mother or ongoing bouts of depression in either parent, may cause this family member to be seen as damaged or abnormal. The impact on the developing child may range from parental absences (emotional or physical), to poor bonding in infancy, modelling difficulties or a lesser capacity of parental involvement during child rearing.

Parental anxiety can lead to hypersensitivity to an infant or young child's somatic responses which, in turn, produce a learned, heightened somatic response in the developing child.

Education

As with many aspects of pain management, education can also assist. Illness (including pain) provides 'opportunities for children to learn about health and illness and to develop strategies for coping with physical discomfort'. An understanding of how learning occurs and how a personality is developed generally, normalises learning and puts the individual (who has perhaps not learned coping behaviours) in the context of learned experiences rather than 'bad behaviour'. A perspective that depersonalises what may otherwise be perceived by parents or the adolescent as blaming for 'bad' behaviour or parenting, is a good place to begin to discuss what and how to change behaviours around pain. Sometimes parents find the opportunity to be less involved a relief, as they already understand that their actions do not change the pain and they feel helpless.

Parents may be more ready than their child to accept their child's independence and self-management techniques for pain. They are likely to be supportive of recommended strategies. It may also be the case that the adolescent is ready to individuate and take steps themself despite their parent's reluctance. An education session with parents and adolescent is part of ongoing assessment as the parents' and adolescent's appraisals and responses to the prospect of independence are likely to become apparent in discussion.

⊶ 'Yellow flags'

Parents who continue to hold a belief that an undiscovered disease or injury is the cause of their child's pain, despite repeated investigations and opinions and despite explanations by their medical practitioners and therapists, are unlikely to accept information presented in pain education as having reference to *their* child. They may have underlying psychopathology perhaps stemming from their own early childhood experiences and that requires longer-term psychotherapy. Such parents may not be in a stage where they will contemplate psychological help (*see* Chapter 4).

Case study: James

James was an immature 12-year-old boy who presented with persistent hip pain of six months' duration. He was the youngest of three children, the two elder children being athletes training at high levels, particularly in tennis. These older children had become annoyed by James's illnesses and the family time they took up. His businessman father was often absent. His mother, a home maker, described James as not 'resilient' like her older children. She described her relationship with James as close, saying he would talk to her about things that he would not tell anyone else. In the assessment they sat very close, his mother looked at him constantly and engaged him in verbal interchanges, touching him frequently. His father sat separately, engaging with James and his wife only briefly at the end.

Jamie's pain was described as sudden in onset following playing tennis and football on the previous day. His referring doctor described a raised erythrocyte sedimentation rate (ESR), suggesting an inflammatory process at the onset of pain. This high reading was never found on later repeated tests. Initially James's mobility deteriorated from being able to use crutches to using a wheelchair. He had missed three months of school. Physiotherapy had apparently made his pain worse. His attempts to walk were characterised by dragging his leg behind him.

A battery of tests revealed no underlying pathology. His mother described that he had had previously an episode of hepatitis secondary to infectious mononucleosis requiring an endoscopy. By the end of the school year, James had progressed to walking normally and had enjoyed a family holiday overseas with lots of walking. The pain recurred on the day before the beginning of the following school year. He attended his first day of school then refused to attend the second, complaining of severe back and hip pain.

It was apparent in assessment that his mother's history recounting was inconsistent. She had failed to report previous recurrent abdominal pain and a history of refusing to attend school when he did not like his teacher. During his bouts of abdominal pain, James missed school, spending his day watching TV at home with his mother. She felt that, as his mother, she could always see when he was 'sick' and unable to go to school. In therapy, it was difficult to achieve regularity of appointments as many were cancelled due to James being unwell with a different source of unwellness each time so that his mother was convinced that her son was ill with other conditions. His mother initiated investigations for a suspected bowel disease and benign hypotension after an optometrist reported swelling behind the eyes. Despite other ophthalmologist specialists agreeing on the normality of the findings, his mother retained a strong sense of uncertainty. No findings of bowel disease were found though James's mother remained unconvinced.

James's function continued to be inconsistent, with his mother remaining anxious and watchful. Despite inconsistent attendance, James learnt some relaxation/mindfulness techniques, which he enjoyed. He found he could lessen intensity and frequency of his new symptoms of headaches and nausea. He had resumed school and had even played some tennis on the weekend. However, his mother felt that he was still unwell and asked to be taught the techniques so that she could do them for him when required. Following a fall in the schoolyard, James missed the following sessions. His mother was 'disappointed' that the school had not called her to inform her of the fall.

She discouraged James from attempting tennis the following day and reported a complete relapse of clinging behaviour, pain, fatigue and poor school attendance following this event.

Comment

This case study highlights the complex interweaving of family relationships (the enmeshed mother and absent father) with medical uncertainties and how these uncertainties exacerbate anxieties and impact on pain and dysfunction. A number of family factors are apparent. James, as the youngest child, with a history of being unwell, was the least naturally athletic, and found himself alienated from his siblings. (One of James's goals was that he wanted a good relationship with his oldest brother!) His mother constructed a story around James's lack of resilience in comparison with that of his siblings. Consequently, she read James's downcast look and non-participation in the siblings' backyard tennis games as evidence only of illness. The mother's 'rescuing' in the name of mothering deprived James of exposure to the necessary experiences of independent coping. His mother described mothering as her 'raison d'être'; she had no apparent other outside interests and James was her last child.

In therapy, time was spent alone with the father. He described his wife as 'fragile' and needing 'black-and-white' answers. The team felt that James's mother perceived any attempts at independent management of pain by James as a threat and that the ongoing 'medical mysteries' caused anxiety for her. In a team meeting with the family, all medical uncertainties were addressed. The family agreed that they would accept whatever the third opinion was from a paediatric ophthalmologist with regard to the benign hypotension, and the third opinion of a paediatrician with regard to the other queries. James's mother wanted to pursue allergies as a source of the abdominal pain. Once these were in place, the family agreed to explore family issues with increasing involvement by the father in his son's activities and a non-pharmacological management plan for James's pain.

References

1 Walker LS, Greene JW. Children with recurrent abdominal pain and their parents: more somatic complaints, anxiety, and depression than other patient families? *J Ped Psychol.* 1989; **14**: 231–4.

2 Bennet SM, Huntsman E, Lilley CM. Parent perceptions of the impact of chronic pain in children and adolescents. *Child Health Care.* 2000; **29**: 147–59.

3 Mechanic C. Adolescent health and illness behaviour: review of the literature and a new hypothesis for study of stress. *J Human Stress.* 1983; **9**: 4–12.

4 Melamed BG, Bush JP. Family factors in children with acute illness. In: Turk DC, Kerns RS, editors. *Health, Illness and Families: a life span perspective.* New York: Wiley; 1985, pp. 183–219.

5 Parmelee AH. Children's illnesses: their beneficial effects on behavioural development. *Child Dev.* 1986; **57**: 1–10.

6 Walker LS, Zeman JL. Parental response to child illness behaviour. *J Ped Psychol.* 1992; **17**(1): 49–71.

7 Bernstein BA, Pachter LM. Cultural considerations in children's pain. In: Schechter N, Berde C, Yaster M, editors. *Pain in Infants, Children, and Adolescents.* Philadelphia: Lippincott Williams & Wilkins; 2003.

8 Zaborowski M. Cultural components in response to pain. *J Social Issues.* 1952; **8**: 16–30.

9 Fordyce W. *Behavioural Methods for Chronic Pain and Illness.* St Louis: Mosby; 1976.

10 Craig K. Modelling and social learning factors in chronic pain. In: Bonica J, editor. *Advances in Pain Research*, vol. 5. New York: Raven, 1983, pp. 813–27.

11 Flor HM, Turk DD, Rudy TE. Relationship of pain impact and significant other reinforcement on pain behaviours: the mediating role of gender, marital status and marital satisfaction. *Pain.* 1989; **38**(1): 45–50.

12 Edwards PW, Zeichner AR, Kuczmierczyk AR. Familial pain models: the relationship between family history of pain and current pain experience. *Pain.* 1995; **21**: 379–84.

13 http://www.bath.ac.uk/pain-management/

14 Flouri E, Buchanan A. The role of father involvement in children's later mental health. *J Adoles.* 2003; **26**: 63–78.

15 Scotford A, Eccleston C, Crombez G. Experiences of fathers of an adolescent with chronic pain. *J Pain.* 2004; **5** (Suppl. 1): 701.

16 Peterson CC, Palermo TM. Parental reinforcement of recurrent pain: the moderating impact of child depression and anxiety on functional disability. *J Ped Psychol.* 2004; **29**(5): 331–41.

17 Dunn-Geier BJ, McGrath PJ, Rourke BP. Adolescent chronic pain: the ability to cope. *Pain.* 1986; **26**: 23–32.

18 Merlijn VPBM, Hunfeld JAM, van der Wouden JC. Psychosocial factors associated with chronic pain in adolescents *Pain.* 2003; **101**(1–2): 33–43.

19 Osborne RB, Hatcher HW, Richtsmeier AJ. The role of social modelling in unexplained paediatric pain. *J Ped Psychol.* 1989; **14**: 43–61.

20 Rickard L. The occurrence of maladaptive health-related behaviours and teacher-rated conduct problems in children of chronic low back pain patients. *J Beh Med.* 1988; **11**: 107–16.

21 Steele RG, Forehand R, Armistead L. Chronic illness and child coping. *J Ab Child Psychol.* 1997; **25**(2): 83–94.

22 Reid GJ, Gilbert CA, McGrath PJ. The Pain Coping Questionnaire: preliminary validation. *Pain.* 1998; **76**: 83–96.

23 Eccleston C, Crombez G, Scotford A, *et al.* Adolescent chronic pain: patterns and predictors of emotional distress in adolescents with chronic pain and their parents. *Pain.* 2004; **108**(3): 221–9.

24 Logan DE, Guite JW, Sherry DD, *et al.* Adolescent-parent relationships in the context of adolescent chronic pain conditions. *Clin J Pain.* 2006; **22**(6): 576–83.

25 Goodman JE, Gidron Y, McGrath PJ. Pain proneness in children: toward a new conceptual framework. In: Grzesiak RC, Ciccone DS, editors. *Psychological Vulnerability to Chronic Pain.* New York: Springer; 1994.

26 Merlijn VPBM, Hunfeld JAM, van der Wouden JC. Psychosocial factors associated with chronic pain in adolescents *Pain.* 2003; **101**(1–2): 33–43.

27 Hatch E. Culture. In: Kuper J, editor. *The Social Science Encyclopedia.* London: Tourledge & Kegan Paul; 1985, pp. 78–179.

28 Bernstein BA, Pachter LM. Cultural considerations in children's pain. In: Schechter N, Berde CB, Yaster M, editors. *Pain in Infants, Children and Adolescents.* Baltimore: Williams & Wilkins; 1993.

29 Jordan AL, Eccleston C, Osborn M. Being a parent of the adolescent with complex chronic pain: an interpretative phenomenological analysis. *Eur J Pain*. 2007; **11**: 49–56.
30 Bandura A, O'Leary A, Barr Taylor C, *et al*. Perceived self-efficacy and pain control: opioid and non-opioid mechanisms. *J Person and Soc Psychol*. 1987; **53**(3): 563–71.
31 Goodman JE, McGrath PJ, Forward SP. Aggregation of pain complaints and pain-related disability and handicap in a community sample of families. In: Jensen TS, Turner JA, Wiesenfeld-Hallen Z, editors. *Progress in Pain Research and Management*, vol. 8. Proceedings of the 8th World Congress on Pain. Seattle: IASP Press; 1997, pp. 673–82.
32 Cano S, Gillis M, Heinz W. Marital functioning, chronic pain, and psychological distress. *Pain*. 2004; **107**(1–2): 167–75.

CHAPTER 4

Sleep

ABOUT SLEEP AND SLEEP HABITS

CHAPTER SUMMARY

This chapter outlines the significant influences and interrelationship between pain and sleep. The characteristics of sleep are described. Assessment of sleep for the individual adolescent is described in respect of factors such as sleep habits, environment, early sleep history, waking habits and sleep-initiation behaviours. The role of the therapist is discussed with suggestions for assisting in the management of night pain and the role of parents. Suggested strategies address preparation for sleep, initiating sleep and changing routines. Reference is made to an earlier case study in which sleep is addressed.

Background

Sleep is one of the first casualties in the individual with chronic or persistent pain. Sleep is necessary for optimal physical and mental functioning in healthy individuals, and is of importance for the body's immune system and healing. It is not simply rest; it is an active process, with some regions of the brain as active during sleep as during wakefulness. Deep sleep is accompanied by deep muscle relaxation with almost complete atonia in the muscles. The transition stage of adolescence is associated with many changes in sleep, including a decrease in duration, delay in the timing of initiating sleep and an increase in the difference between weekday and weekend sleep patterns.[1,2,3] Up to 16% of adolescents have clinically significant insomnia.[4,5,6] Insufficient sleep is associated with a vicious cycle of short- and long-term negative effects on mood, self-control of emotions and attention, diminished motivation, increased school absences and difficulties with concentration and academic performance.[7,8,9] Disturbed sleep in adolescents with persistent pain has been associated with significant impairments in a range of physical and social activities along with reductions in overall health-related quality of life.[10]

Between 50% and 65% of children and adolescents who have chronic pain have sleep disturbance.[11] Most commonly, adolescents with persistent pain describe difficulties initiating sleep, frequent waking and excessive daytime sleepiness. Several studies of adults and children report poor sleep associated with increase in pain.[12,13,14] It is likely that the relationship between pain and sleep is bi-directional with pain disrupting sleep and poor sleep increasing pain sensitivity.[15,16] The relationship between pain and sleep is further complicated by the high incidence of co-morbid psychological disorders such as anxiety and depression and some chronic pain conditions, including recurrent abdominal pain and fibromyalgia, that are also characterised by poor sleep.[17,18]

Sleep

Two states of sleep, rapid eye movement (REM) sleep (sometimes described as deep sleep) and non-REM, involve two distinct neural pathways. REM sleep is characterised by deep muscle relaxation with almost complete atonia in the muscles, high cortical function associated with dreaming and bursts of rapid eye movement. Non-REM sleep is characterised by relatively low brain activity and some body movements. Non-REM sleep has four separate stages. Continuity, timing and patterning of the different stages, including transition from REM to non-REM, are necessary for restorative sleep. Night waking results in increased secretion of cortisol, the hormone associated with increased stress, while sleep onset is associated with suppression of cortisol release.[19] An adolescent with pain, waking several times a night, will be interrupting this process and will report fatigue and mood changes.

There is a close link between sleep and perceptions of safety and threat. As sleep is a state that involves a loss of consciousness of, and responsiveness to, the environment, most animals have evolved mechanisms to ensure sleep behaviours are limited to safe places. Where an individual does not feel safe, they do not want to turn off vigilance and responsiveness, leading to a state of alertness at onset of sleep. 'Bedtime rituals and sleep onset associations are also extremely powerful and are linked to threat and arousal systems. Strong and problematic associations may develop between bedtime fears of separation, being alone, worry about illness and physical sensations of pain'.[20,21]

There may be a number of factors that add to the state of alertness at the time of onset of sleep for the adolescent with pain, as listed below.

- Pain sensations activate a threat-related arousal state, with heightened vigilance to signals for the onset of pain.
- Pain signals activate the memory and cognitive areas of the cerebral cortex, causing affective disturbances. In other words, pain may initiate thoughts about loss, blame or threat, in turn leading to feelings of depression, anger or worry. (*See* Chapter 1.)
- Separation issues, with associated fears learned from early childhood, are likely to manifest at bedtime when the adolescent is alone. Inability to initiate sleep onset may be a longstanding problem.
- Parents may have their own separation issues, fearing a loss of vigilance to their child's pain. A parent's anxiety perceived by the child may in turn reinforce any anxiety in the adolescent.

A relationship exists between anxiety and pain. Adolescents with chronic pain identify more fears of failure and experiences of less social acceptance.[22] Adolescents unable to initiate sleep have more time to worry about a range of psychosocial factors that occur for them. Worry, in turn, exacerbates their state of alertness and so maintains the vicious cycle of sleep difficulty and thoughts about their inability to cope the next day.

Assessment

Asking the following questions may provide information that is useful in assessing sleep difficulties:

- What does the adolescent report as their main problem?
- What is the parent's perception of the main problem (a) for them as the parent, and (b) for their child?

Sleep habits and pattern

- Is the main difficulty getting off to sleep or staying asleep?
- What time do they get into bed? Is it roughly the same time every night and is there a time difference between when they go to sleep on weekends from during the week for a school/work night?
- Do they take coffee, tea or other drugs within approximately four hours before going to sleep?

⊃ How many times do they wake at night? What wakes them: pain, restlessness, worry, temperature, noise?

⊃ What do they do when they wake, e.g. turn on the light, get up and read, eat, watch TV, worry, call their parent? How long before they are they able to put themselves back to sleep?

⊃ If a parent comes in, what do they do – massage, get a heat pack, medication, console, sit with them?

⊃ Does the parent hear them grinding their teeth, snoring, crying or getting up?

⊃ Do they do anything else in bed prior to attempting to go to sleep, e.g. read for a long time, watch TV, listen to rock music or talk to a friend on the phone?

⊃ What time do they wake up in the morning? Who wakes them?

⊃ How much exercise do they get during the day?

⊃ Do they lie down or sleep during the day?

Environment

⊃ Where do they sleep – in their own room, with other siblings, in their parents' room or bed?

⊃ Do they have a TV in their room?

⊃ Is noise a factor?

History

⊃ What was the adolescent's sleeping pattern prior to the onset of the pain, including in early childhood?

With these details it is possible to get a picture of the problems that can be addressed with help. Educating the adolescent and parent about sleep hygiene is a good way to begin. During this discussion it will be apparent whether the parent has been able to provide bedtime structure in the past and whether they have any influence over bed routine at the present time. Problems with bladder or bowel, snoring or tooth grinding need specific referral to the appropriate medical or dental practitioner.

Having sufficient information allows a good formulation of the nature of the individual adolescent's sleep problem. What may seem like a single problem, such as initiating sleep, may have multiple causes and several different solutions. Helping the adolescent to solve stress inducing problems may involve family therapy, school contact, social workers, etc.

Initiating sleep onset

Difficulty in initiating sleep onset may be the result of:

⊃ an old habit carried over from early childhood where no consistent bedtime rituals were established or where sleep was only ever initiated with the help of a parent (now, in adolescence, perhaps with the aid of a TV in the room)

⊃ generalised anxiety, or anxiety about coping while being tired and in pain, or worry about a specific problem such as bullying, academic performance, the meaning of the pain, parental discord, etc.
⊃ increased awareness of pain
⊃ insufficient exercise in the day or napping during the day
⊃ intake of caffeine or other stimulants in the evening.

Frequent or early waking
Frequent or early waking may be the result of:
⊃ pain awareness
⊃ sensitivity to noise, light or parental activity
⊃ insufficient exercise the previous day
⊃ too much fluid intake just prior to going to bed.

Inability to get back to sleep after waking
Inability to get back to sleep after waking may be the result of:
⊃ rewards in the environment such as parental or sibling attention
⊃ hyper-alertness
⊃ anxiety
⊃ pain
⊃ poor habits such as eating, intake of drugs (including caffeine), or watching TV late at night; phoning friends.

Diagnostic criteria
There are diagnostic criteria for insomnia. A psychologist will assist in discriminating between primary sleep disorders and sleep disorders related to other mental disorders such as depression or anxiety.

Treatment
Treatment may include any of the following.
⊃ Drug treatment. Although other drugs exist for sleep, in pain clinics a commonly used drug to assist with sleep and pain is very low doses of the anti-depressant amitriptyline. This assists in the initiation and maintenance of sleep. Some adolescents experience a side effect of drowsiness in the morning.
⊃ Sleep hygiene: advice on exercise, naps, food, drugs, clock watching, etc (see below).
⊃ Relaxation-based anxiety reduction and muscle relaxation.
⊃ Stimulus-control procedures based on behavioural learning models – looking at the learning and what maintains it. This requires planning and discipline from the adolescent and entails gradually establishing new patterns of sleep.
⊃ Paradoxical intention, which aims to remove the anxiety of trying to

sleep. This involves purposely keeping the eyes open for as long as possible and congratulating oneself on maintaining open eyes. This is only appropriate only for adolescents with sleep *performance* anxiety.

Referral to a sleep clinic

An adolescent with longstanding sleep problems may need an analysis of their sleep patterns to assist with identifying problems. Polysomnography is the 'gold standard' for assessing physiological sleep.

Changing a habit where the adolescent has lost the distinction between day and night and is sleeping in until the middle of the day or afternoon can be difficult to manage with a home-based programme. These young people may benefit from referral to a sleep clinic where a normal night-and-day pattern can be established. This may entail a similar strategy that is used for jetlag, where the individual is kept awake during the time in the day when they would normally sleep then allowed to sleep at the appropriate time the following night. Keeping someone awake for a whole night can be more than a family can manage at home (especially if parents need to work and if the adolescent is very grumpy, being sleep deprived).

Sleep apnoea may also indicate the need for a sleep clinic referral.

The role of the therapist with the adolescent

Most adolescents need support in the process of organising themselves in a new way or to change habits. Having a person who is not their parent to help them gives a sense of independence and coping.

A session explaining the learned nature of sleep is advisable so that the adolescent understands that they are retraining their body. Emphasise that change can be slow. Work out the cause of the sleep difficulty with the adolescent targeting the problem and working through solutions that are effective for that individual.

Ask at the beginning of each session for the positive changes first off; this it is a way of focussing on success rather than on the problems.

Follow up and assess the success of home practice of any suggestions.

Setting baselines can help, although these rely essentially on subjective recording and can be unreliable. A more objective measure is actigraphy which records body movements and estimates sleep and wake states – it involves wearing a watch-like device.[23] If this is unavailable, initially keep a record of times of going to bed, onset of sleep and hours of sleep (perhaps observed by a parent) so as to measure progress by comparing this with a later recording, e.g. in a few weeks' or months' time. (*See* Chapter 5.) Remember that after this initial recording, clock watching is not advised.

See **Case study: Angela (Chapter 3).**

O⊸ 'Yellow flags'

Night pain

Parents who have been living with a child whose pain has been out of control during the night can feel fatigued and at their wits' end. They are, at the same time, likely to be extra vigilant to their child's sounds and behaviours in response to pain. They may strongly believe that their child cannot cope alone because their behaviour has shown this, and believe that their child will feel abandoned if left alone to cope.

⊃ Discuss with both parties whether the parent's presence changes the pain level. (I have never heard an adolescent report that the presence of their parent actually results in less pain.)

⊃ Having established this, a discussion about the benefits of independent managing can be useful. Refer back to valued activities and goals, i.e. the adolescent can stay over at friends' houses or go on camp; the parent gets more sleep, etc.

⊃ Separate management of anxiety or depressive symptoms may be necessary.

⊃ Suggest trialling the process for a prescribed time, e.g. three months.

⊃ Start the adolescent with strategies to manage negative body sensations – including pain. They will need to practise independently and *as soon as possible* so that they feel equipped with some action to take. (*See* Chapter 7.)

Working with the parent

Usually parents acknowledge their frustration and inability to relieve pain. Having established that they are unable to take the pain away and that independent coping is desirable, suggest a gradual change of parent behaviour.

⊃ If the adolescent has been in the parental bed, start a jointly agreed reward-based programme (*see* Chapter 5), i.e. sleeping in their own bed for a number of nights earns an agreed reward – for a whole term, a larger one again (perhaps this one as a reward for final achievement).

⊃ If the parent is in the habit of going into the bedroom when the adolescent calls out, commence a gradually increasing delay of entry to their bedroom to allow time for the adolescent to apply independent strategies.

⊃ Suggest that the parent can endorse their child's coping by always asking what the adolescent has done for themselves (relaxation, visualisation). Remind the parent that their attention to their child is a reward, so they need to be aware that they are rewarding their child's independent effort, not their inability to sleep.

⊃ Propose a slow, gradual withdrawal of parental attention for parents worried they may be abandoning or repressing their child. This gradual success is, in itself, convincing that no harm is coming to their child, especially as everyone begins to reap the benefits of better sleep.
A reward-based programme for fewer calls by the adolescent to the

parent may work if parents are convinced of 'no harm', as mentioned above.

The handout 'Strategies for sleep' incorporates many suggestions for managing a multiplicity of sleep problems (*see also* Handout 1 in the Appendix). The handout is best used when tailored to the individual's needs. Remove any suggestions irrelevant to their circumstances. So it would be advisable to choose which suggestions target the specific problem the individual adolescent is experiencing. For instance, an active adolescent having difficulty sleeping because of worries may not need suggestions relating to sufficient exercise. Leaving this in may even cause an impatient or frustrated adolescent to perceive the handout as generally irrelevant, thereby rejecting the other more relevant points. A few simple, well-targeted suggestions are much more likely to be read and applied. After modifying the handout, suggest the adolescent fixes it to their wall or near their bed. Always go through each suggestion in the handout to make sure they are clear.

All sleep difficulties will be assisted with the teaching of basic relaxation techniques (*see* Chapter 7). It is important to teach these independent of relaxation tapes because these tapes may not always be available, for instance whilst staying over at a friend's house.

Strategies for sleep

These strategies have been found to be very useful in assisting people to sleep. They can be particularly helpful if you are experiencing pain which interferes with your sleep.

Preparing for sleep
⊃ **Establish a routine.** If you go to bed at the same time every night, you are training your body to know when it should be ready to sleep. No matter how much sleep you have had, try to get up at the same time in the morning. Use an alarm clock for this. The body needs to experience hours of daylight in order to distinguish night from day, which triggers the message for sleep.
⊃ **Keep to the routine even on weekends and holidays** if you are training yourself to establish a routine. You need to do this at least for a few months until your sleep habits are established. Staying up until after midnight will trigger the old learned habits of sleep difficulty. You may be able to sleep in, once you have retrained your body into the new habits for a sufficient period of time.
⊃ **Sleeping in the daytime is not a good idea** as this confuses your body clock, and makes it more difficult to sleep at night.
⊃ **Do some physical exercise during the day** (walking is especially good). This means you are physically, not just mentally, tired at the end of the day.

➲ **Avoid stimulants in the evenings**, e.g. drinking caffeine or alcohol. These inhibit getting to sleep. Instead, a small warm milk drink or herbal tea can help you to settle to sleep. You may have a light snack.

➲ **Keep your bed as a place for sleep, not anything else.** When you get into bed, say to yourself, 'Now I am going to sleep.' It is not a good idea to watch TV, talk on the phone, or do homework in bed. If you keep your bed for sleeping only, your body gets the message that when you get into bed it is time for sleep.

➲ **If you are unable to sleep after 10–15 minutes, get out of bed**, go to another room and do a quiet activity until you feel sleepy, then begin again. You may need to do this several times to start with.

➲ **Avoid stimulating activities near bedtime** such as exercise, having stimulating chats or arguments, eating heavy meals (a light snack is OK), or doing demanding intellectual work. Give yourself wind-down time. Calming activities that can help some people settle to sleep include: reading a book or magazine, listening to easy music or the radio, having a warm (not too hot) bath or shower. Try to notice any signs of tiredness in your body, as this is the best time to go to bed.

➲ **Use the relaxation strategies** you have learnt before you get into bed, or if you wake up during the night. Focus your mind and use breathing or mindfulness techniques to let go of any worries. Although this focus may seem difficult to start at night, it can be surprisingly more effective, especially if you have been practising at other times. If focus seems especially hard, limit yourself to 10 or 20 breaths to start. Mark these off by moving a finger with each breath. Don't use numbers to count, as this is distracting from the focus on breath. This is helpful in the middle of the night to assist getting back to sleep.

➲ **Use your imagination positively.** This is like creating your own movie (or dream) behind your eyes. Imagine a quiet place or activity you love, fill in all the physical details including colour texture and smell of the place. Put yourself in this movie and freely move about. The place or activity you create can be whatever or wherever you want, in the country, by the sea, at home – what matters is that it is peaceful and feels safe and interesting to you.

➲ **Keep a notebook by the bed**, so if your thoughts are racing or worrying, you can write them down. Tell yourself that it is unlikely that you will find a solution right now and that your mind is just on repetititive 'tram tracks'. It's OK to stop thinking about them now because you can think about them in the morning when you are more likely to find a solution.

Remember

➲ If you don't sleep tell yourself it is OK. Whilst lying in bed your body is resting and you will be all right in the morning.

➲ Make sure clock faces are not visible so that you are not 'clock watching'.

➲ A routine may take several months of persistent practice to establish.

➲ In general, no harm will occur if you do not sleep for one or two nights. Remember you are still resting and you will catch up on sleep later because you are tired.

➲ Accept that progress may be slow, especially if the problem has been there a while. If it seems hard and you are losing heart, keep a log of your sleeping patterns and compare them with your earlier baseline. You can gradually move your going-to-bed time back by 15 minutes at a time for a week or so. To keep yourself on track, record whatever factors are affecting your sleep, such as difficulty getting to sleep, how long you slept for, how many times you woke in the night, and how you felt when waking up in the morning.

➲ If sleep issues or pain are extreme or continue to get worse, you may benefit from visiting a sleep clinic or discussing with your pain specialist doctor pain medications that can also assist sleep. But remember that medications are only a short-term answer, retraining yourself is the long-term solution.

Changing routine to an earlier time

It is common for adolescents who have been away from school for a prolonged period to have turned day into night by sleeping until midday or later, then being unable to sleep until the hours after midnight.

This usually arises because the adolescent with pain becomes more aware of pain in bed and has difficulty initiating sleep and so avoids it. A vicious cycle of fatigue then ensues. If the problem has arisen as a result of attempting to control persistent pain, i.e. if it is not a life pattern, it may be possible to move these times forward over a period of time.

Holiday periods are the best for this as prolonging time away from school is not recommended while adjustment is made. Frequently sleep patterns slip over long holiday times. If parents are at work the adolescent gradually increases their sleeping-in habits. It is advisable to tackle this problem well before the end of holidays to give adjustment time. Values-based work and commitment to actions that are in those directions can help in ownership of the process.

Establish a baseline of when the adolescent is retiring to bed.

Decide on a time of waking that they feel they will be able to achieve and that is within range of a normal time to rise. Use an alarm clock (not a parent) for this. This waking time must be rigidly adhered to.

Gradually move the time of going to bed earlier by 15 minutes, increasing this over days as sleep is achieved. Use relaxation, visualisation, etc. to support this. As the time to sleep changes, revise the waking time accordingly until the desired time is achieved. It does not hurt to have days of fatigue if the time of waking is radically moved forward. This is how most adolescents without pain make the change from holiday time to school time.

References

1 Iglowsein I, Jenni OG, Lolinari L, *et al.* Sleep duration from infancy to adolescence: reference values and generational trends. *Pediatrics.* 2003; **111**: 302–7.

2 Carskadon MA, Wolfson AR, Acebo C, *et al.* Adolescent sleep patterns, circadian timing, and sleepiness at a transition to early school days. *Sleep.* 1998; **21**: 871–81.

3 Wolfson AR, Carskadon MA. Sleep schedules and daytime functioning in adolescents. *Child Dev.* 1998; **69**: 875–7.

4 Morrison DN, McGee R, Stanton WR. Sleep problems in adolescence. *J Acad Child Adolesc Psychiatry.* 1992; **31**: 94–9.

5 Ohayon MM, Caulet M, Lemoine P. Comorbidity of mental and insomnia disorders in the general population. *Compr Psychiatry.* 1998; **39**: 185–97.

6 Roberts RE, Lee ES, Hemandez M, *et al.* Symptoms of insomnia among adolescents in the lower Rio Grande Valley of Texas. *Sleep.* 2004; **27**: 751–60.

7 Fallone G, Owens JA, Deane J. Sleepiness in children and adolescents: clinical implications. *Sleep Med Rev.* 2002; **6**: 287–386.

8 Bonnet M. Sleep deprivation. In: Kyger MH, Roth T, Dement WC, editors. *Principles and Practice of Sleep Medicine.* Philadelphia, PA: WB Saunders; 1994.

9 Pearlman CA. Sleep structure variation and performance. In: Webb WB, editor. *Biological Rhythms, Sleep and Performance.* New York: John Wiley and Sons; 1982.

10 Palermo TM, Kiska R. Subjective sleep disturbances in adolescents with chronic pain: relationship to daily functioning and quality of life. *J Pain.* 2005; **6**: 201–7.

11 Roth-Isigeit A, Thyen U, Stoven H. Pain among children and adolescents: restrictions in daily living. *Paediatrics.* 2005; **115**(2): e152–e162.

12 Wilson KG, Watson ST, Currie SR. Daily diary and ambulatory activity monitoring of sleep in patients with insomnia associated with chronic musculoskeletal pain. *Pain.* 1998; **75**: 75–84.

13 McCracken LM, Iverson GL. Pain. *Pain Res Manag.* 2002; **7**(2): 75–9.

14 Bruni O, Gabrizi P, Ottaviano S, *et al.* Prevalence of sleep disorders in childhood and adolescence with headache: a case-control study. *Cephalalgia.* 1997; **17**: 492–8.

15 Lewin DS, Dahl RE. Importance of sleep in the management of pediatric pain. *J Dev Behav Ped.* 1999; **20**: 244–52.

16 Palermo TM. Impact of recurrent and chronic pain in child and family daily functioning: a critical review of the literature. *J Dev Behav Ped.* 2000; **21**: 58–69.

17 Walker LS, Guite JW, Duke M, *et al.* Recurrent abdominal pain: a potential precursor of irritable bowel syndrome in adolescents and young adults. *J Pediatr.* 1998; **132**: 1010–5.

18 Hyams JS. Recurrent abdominal pain and irritable bowel syndrome in children. *J Pediatr Gastoenterol Nutr.* 1997; **25**(1): 16–7.

19 Davidson KR, Moldofsky H, Lue FA. Growth hormone and cortisol secretion in relation to sleep wakefulness. *J Psychiat Neurosci.* 1991; **16**: 96–102.

20 Lewin DS, Dahl RW. Importance of sleep in the management of pediatric pain. *Devel and Beh Pediatr.* 1999; **20**(4): 244–52.

21 Ferber R. *Solve Your Child's Sleep Problems.* New York: Simon & Schuster; 1985.

22 Merlijn VPBM, Hunnfeld JAM, van der Wouden JC, *et al.* Psychosocial factors associated with chronic pain in adolescents. *Pain.* 2003; **101**(1–2): 33–43.

23 Ankoli-Israel S, Cole R, Alessi C, *et al.* The role of actigraphy in the study of sleep and circadian rhythms. *Sleep.* 2003; **26**: 342–92.

CHAPTER 5

Making changes

ABOUT VALUES, GOALS AND MOTIVATION

CHAPTER SUMMARY

This chapter discusses how to change the agenda of the adolescent and family from pain control to restoration of a fulfilling life. It looks at what motivates change. It suggests a cost/benefit discussion and how to access the adolescent's values and goals as primary motivators. Steps in this process are identified. How to recognise resistance in therapy is described with suggestions for its management. There is discussion on different forms of goal setting and associated processes. Measures presented include the use of the Canadian Occupational Performance Measure (COPM), the Goal Attainment Scale (GAS) and Target Complaints. An example case study incorporates the use of COPM.

Background

Usually, families and adolescents feel they have made many attempts to 'fix' the problem and despite having done all they can, they have been unsuccessful. They feel ineffective. For these adolescents and families, the cost has been high. They feel 'stuck' and with no imaginable forward direction. Suggesting change can therefore feel like suggesting the impossible. It can also offer hope as it suggests a future where there seemed to be none. It can feel challenging and scary because the parent and adolescent do not feel capable of action and/or because change will cause them to face emotions or events they have avoided, in the interests of avoiding pain. For these people, avoidance is an attempt to remain in control. A developmental history and case formulation (*see* 'Assessment' in Chapter 1) will identify what sort of change may provoke threat and anxiety in the adolescent or their parent. Exposure to these threats needs to be managed consciously and in a graduated way.

Changing the agenda from pain control

In the initial assessment, asking what has been tried in order to control the pain is an important question that will identify the adolescent's and family's agenda for therapy. Additionally, it is useful to ask what it is that the adolescent or parent expects from seeking help. It may be that they request assistance with 'managing' the pain. Others want 'the pain to go away'; others may say 'I want my life back.' While these seem to represent different expectations, the adolescent's or parent's underlying assumption is likely to be to remove, diminish or control the pain before they can feel capable or motivated to change. Only if they can 'control' the pain or only if the pain is less do they feel they can start to move forward. This may not be overtly acknowledged; however, it is implicit in their inability to progress up to this point. Their attempts at controlling, diminishing or removing the pain up to this point have involved attempting to avoid situations that elicit the pain (exercise, school or socialising), and possibly other, unpleasant experiences such as anxiety. The cost of their attempts has been high and yet the unpleasant experience remains.

Motivation to change

The effort to understand what motivates some people to persist in the face of adversity (in this case, persistent or chronic pain), has occupied many researchers. In college students with persistent pain, the *enjoyment* of goal pursuit suffers while evaluative dampening or goal 'degeneration' is also associated with pain.[1] Motivational enhancement therapy (MET) first postulated that changing addictive behaviours in adults is based on four stages of change: precontemplation, contemplation, action and maintenance. This theory proposes that adults in different states of change demonstrate different success rates and *require different treatment strategies appropriate to their stage of change.*[2] Developments on this theory for adult pain patients have resulted in attempts to measure the construct of stages and forward movement from one stage to another. Primarily this measure was proposed to predict outcomes of treatment. In a review of the literature, it was suggested that the four stages were better represented as two: contemplation and engagement.[3] Self-efficacy was of greater predictive value for adults with chronic pain in determining treatment outcomes.[4]

The Multidimensional Pain Readiness to Change Questionnaire has attempted to address the multifactorial aspects within a multidisciplinary adult pain-management programme.[5,6] These aspects include exercise, relaxation, cognitive strategies, pacing, and assertive communication. The individual may be in a different stage of readiness to change with each of these aspects of a programme. For instance, they may be open to cognitive strategies but not to exercise. In the absence of measures designed specifically for adolescents, the need to consider readiness for change remains, in order to avoid ineffective therapeutic techniques, resistance to treatment and treatment failure resulting in disappointment, further frustration and even anger. In the adolescent population, assessment must also include parental readiness to change as a separate entity.

Contextual cognitive behavioural therapy (CCBT) and acceptance commitment therapy (ACT) (*see* Introduction) describe the process as one of willingness to accept the negative private events of pain, unwanted thoughts and emotions that have often been the object of avoidance. Willingness and acceptance lead to change because the individual can make decisions that are not driven by efforts to avoid having the negative private events. It frees the individual from the struggle and allows different choices for actions that are personally meaningful, derived from the individual's values and which result in increasing patterns of new learning with rewarding outcomes.

A short questionnaire (20 items) that approaches the question of motivation from the perspective of willingness to engage in life activities while accepting pain (rather than avoiding it) is the Chronic Pain Acceptance Questionnaire.[7]

A manual of acceptance commitment therapy for adolescents has been developed by Laurie Greco, based on the work of Steven Hayes. It describes 10 sessions with exercises specifically dealing with the areas outlined below. This manual is most suitable for group work.[8,9]

A cost/benefit discussion

It is important to ask what has already changed for the adolescent and family since the presence of persistent pain. Placing at centre stage the present state of their life in a discussion can be confronting and upsetting for them. Some adolescents have not wanted to contemplate this overview of their situation, because they will feel sad or a failure. The negative emotions or thoughts generated by this discussion may be internal events also avoided by the adolescent. Acknowledging their existence at this point is important as it leads naturally into a discussion about the possibility that negative emotions might arise in the therapy process to follow. Asking for effort and commitment is part of this process and is a useful preparation. At this point (of facing the difficulties) the therapist might ask the adolescent as part of their observation of the adolescent's process – 'Am I correct in thinking that this hard for you?' 'Is this one of those difficult times we talked about before?' Consent by the adolescent to accept difficulty as part of the process is a beginning of willingness in therapy and is a positive step even at this early stage. Reflect this first positive step back to the adolescent if they agree to continue. It also makes discussion and acceptance of difficult emotions part of the process to come.

It is also a useful discussion to have with the parent, as they, too, need to consent to a degree of unpleasant, sometimes challenging, feelings in observing their child's efforts, discomfort, and pain. They, too, may have been avoiding in the same way.

Cost/benefit questions that may help are:
- ⊃ 'What has the pain cost so far?'
- ⊃ 'What have you had to stop doing?'
- ⊃ 'What have you tried to do to fix this?
- ⊃ 'What has worked for you?' (They may at this point describe how massage or heat packs work for them; it is best not to argue against such coping strategies, but rather to simply accept the adolescent's perspective.)
- ⊃ 'Is the problem (the pain or other) still there despite what you have tried?' (There may be other problems identified as part of the negative experiences – anxiety, bullying, academic or social failure.)
- ⊃ 'What would life look like if a magic wand made the pain and all other identified problems disappear?'
- ⊃ 'What are the potential benefits of doing things while still experiencing pain?'

Understanding the adolescent's view of an idealised life without pain allows a comparison to be made between what they rationalise as working and what is actually not working. In doing this, the therapist is beginning to identify, in conjunction with the adolescent, what sort of young person they would like to be. This is an opening to a discussion about their values.

Values and goals as motivators

Values are what give *meaning* to a person's life. Values are essentially neutral, neither right nor wrong: they simple 'are'. They are something you move towards rather than achieve, as a goal is achieved. A useful image is that a value is like a point on the horizon that you never reach though you constantly aim for it and refer to it as a guide. In a healthy individual, actions and decisions on behaviours are first unconsciously referenced according to 'fit' with the individual's values. ('Is this a good thing to do?') Goals are the tangible events on the journey to the point on the horizon. Goals which are achievable act like signposts on the journey. Value-driven behaviour change is more likely to be sustained over time than goal-driven behaviour change.

The mesolimbic area of the brain is the area associated with rewards (*see* Chapter 1) and decisions to take action in a reward-based direction, i.e. making quick money as in the case of compulsive gamblers, releases endogenous opioids (i.e. the pleasure taken in gambling).[10] This same area is also active in the neurophysiological processing of pain. It is hypothesised that if a person chooses to behave in a way that will produce a valued reward, the body's natural painkillers are released. An example may be of an academic who has a headache and who is in the middle of writing a submission for ongoing funding that will ensure his/her employment in his/her *valued* area of research. If there is a short time frame for this submission and the academic chooses to continue despite the headache, it is postulated that opioids will be released and the headache will lessen (*see* Chapter 1).

Identifying values

After first clarifying that the adolescent understands the concept of a value, draw up a picture or diagram of how they would like others to describe them. This may be a difficult concept to convey initially. It may help to describe it in metaphors. For example, what would they like people (friends/teachers/family) to say about them? Imagine a going-away party, a write-up of themselves in the paper, or perhaps speeches made at a 21st birthday party. In other words, what would they like their life to stand for?

Ask the adolescent:
⊃ 'How do you want others to see you?'
⊃ 'What would you like your life to stand for?'

It helps to define domains of an adolescent's life:
⊃ health and physical well-being
⊃ friendships
⊃ recreational activity
⊃ intimate relations (boyfriend/girlfriend)
⊃ family relationships
⊃ spirituality
⊃ school, learning or training
⊃ occupation or work.

This can be done using diagrams of concentric circles starting with the most valued area at the centre, or perhaps in a shape defined by the adolescent – a heart shape can help with the idea of values as being a direction in which the heart leads. Work with the adolescent to elaborate on the details of what life would look like without pain (or other problems) in all domains of their life. This can be further refined in terms of goals.

'Being' and 'doing' goals

If the concept of values is too difficult, a hierarchy of goals can be constructed in terms of *'be'* goals ('How would you like to be?' or 'What sort of person would you like to be?'). These are longer-term ones for which there may be several paths. Shorter-term goals are more *'do'* goals ('What do you want to do?'). 'Do' goals still need to be broken down into a hierarchy of priority and difficulty. The hierarchy may be based on degree of difficulty in facing the fear or anxiety associated with moving towards them (as in graduated exposure therapy). Goals that are *'do'* goals may lead to *'be'* goals in the longer term.

Asking adolescents whether their current actions are taking them closer or further away from their valued direction can be an enlightening thought for them and can assist in their awareness that they want to make different choices of action, i.e. values-based action, despite the existence of pain. This can be the beginning of a commitment to change and a shift from contemplation of change to engagement.

Steps in the process

1 **Engage the adolescent in a relationship.**
   Adolescent is asking:
   ⊃ 'Is this for me? Are they listening to me?'
   ⊃ 'Do I like the therapists?'
   ⊃ 'Will they hurt me?'
   ⊃ 'Can I trust them?'

   Parent is asking:
   ⊃ 'Are they hearing my story?'
   ⊃ 'Will they leave me out? What is my role?'
   ⊃ 'Can I accept the emotions that will accompany changes?'

   Therapist's actions:
   ⊃ Hear the full story.
   ⊃ What has worked, what hasn't worked?
   ⊃ What does the adolescent expect from therapy?
   ⊃ What does the parent expect from therapy?
   ⊃ Reinterpret the agenda from control of pain to fulfilment and enjoyment of life.
2 **Cost versus benefits discussion as presented previously.**
3 **Introduce values-based work** with the adolescent. (This can also be done with the parent with regard to their child. Their values do not need to be in agreement.)

Acknowledge that pain can be difficult to manage. Ask if there have been other difficult things that they have managed? (Draw out whatever particular assets were required here: bravery, commitment, independence, etc.)

4 **Physiology of pain education** with follow-up suggestions for parental role.

5 **Goal setting.**

If the parent or child is in agreement and willing to some degree to participate in at least some of the programme offered, it is possible they have proceeded from pre-contemplation into action.

Offer concrete actions in appropriate areas. (*See* Chapters 3, 4, 8, 7, 9 and 10.)

> •*A therapist who takes action 'for' the adolescent can diminish the adolescent's responsibility for action in the same way as a parent can.*•

⌾ᴫ 'Yellow flag': Resistance

Recognising resistance

Resistance is described as interrupting, arguing, and side-tracking or defensive responding.[11] In the context of adolescent behaviour resistance may take the form of inappropriate merriment, chaotic or excessive 'good ideas' that divert attention, or continual 'Yes, but . . .' responses. In addition, there may be frequent appointment cancellation with plausible excuses (often supported by the parent), failure to carry out actions agreed to with plausible excuses (home practice not executed, homework book forgotten).

Resistance to this change or a lack of willingness can occur if any party feels coerced. It is unlikely the pre-contemplating adolescent or parent will respond to practical suggestions that are the characteristic of an action or engaged stage. It is easy to view the adolescent or parent as 'uncooperative' at this point! By asking questions or reflecting back observations, it is possible to redirect therapy. Questions help if, by answering them, the adolescent or parent finds themself beginning to identify and elucidate problems they wish to overcome, or bringing their current behaviour into doubt. These responses need to be reflected back to the parent or adolescent as they are observed. It may require a revisit of the cost/benefit discussion.

If you find yourself as a therapist in an argument with the adolescent or parent, there is a misjudgement of the stage from which the adolescent or parent is operating. If this occurs, new strategies are necessary, such as:

⊃ shift focus away from the point of the argument

⊃ reflect back in such a way that the adolescent or parent may query the logic or inconsistency of their current position

⊃ roll with resistance by reframing it in different language

⊃ show that you, the therapist, understand that the adolescent (or parent) is finding the change hard[12]

⊃ refer to the initial discussion regarding difficulty and commitment in the process of therapy, and ask if their current behaviour takes them closer or further away from their values.

What makes therapy progress?

1   A parent who wants some changes, even though the adolescent with general anxiety and school avoidance finds it too difficult to contemplate.

2   A change in the parent–child relationship. The appropriateness and degree of parental involvement can play a pivotal role in the outcome for the adolescent. This may mean withdrawal of parental involvement in taking action *for* their child (*see* 'Do's and don'ts' in Chapter 8). For others it may mean a different sort of involvement – such as parents rewarding different behaviour in their child (values-based or goal-based actions); placing of new expectations, rules and boundaries around their child's behaviour; or increasing non-pain-related time with their child. (Chapter 6 describes in more detail issues for parents.)

3   An adolescent at a different stage of change from their parent may choose to move into action independently of their parent and may require support in this process. This may result from a values-based discussion in which they commit to values-based actions. They may choose not to discuss pain with a parent who remains in a pre-contemplation stage, still believing that their child needs their help. It may also be that the adolescent understands the limitation of their parent and decides to work within the bounds of what is possible in their family.

An example of change

Find an example of a daily task such as cutting meat and writing with the right hand. Ask the adolescent to imagine how they would feel if, for one whole day, they were required to have their dominant hand out of action and tied up so that they had to rely on their non-dominant hand. The task chosen should be difficult. If non-dominant hand use is not difficult, work with them to find some task they would find difficult to sustain. They may enjoy actually trying this out for themselves. Common reactions to this exercise are:

⊃ 'It feels strange and clumsy. I feel stupid!'

⊃ 'I'm not used to it, it's uncomfortable!'

⊃ 'I wish I could go back to how I used to do things!'

⊃ 'I can't do it properly. I have to think about it all the time!'

⊃ 'I get tired of it (and may even untie my good hand to give myself a rest from the effort!)'
⊃ 'I don't feel like myself!'

Suggest that if the adolescent has developed a habit, they may experience some of these reactions. These reactions may occur if the parent and adolescent change their behaviour towards each other; for example, a parent not responding with an offer of massage, the adolescent not complaining about pain. This example follows naturally on from the education session about how we learn and the do's and don'ts for parents (*see* Chapters 1 and 3).

Goals

Setting achievable goals is a natural direction that follows values work. It clarifies direction and can be a way of noting change and progress. Asking what they would be doing, what they would look like, how they would be acting if they were choosing to act in the direction of their values can begin this process. Some understanding of actions the adolescent can take in the face of pain (*see* Chapter 9) and awareness of their responses to past experiences, memories or fears (*see* Chapter 7) helps to choose values-based actions.

Why set goals?
⊃ Goals can simplify or direct therapy in an agreed way or can place reasonable limits on outcomes.
⊃ They can be part of a conscious process of graduated exposure to objects of threat (e.g. the thought of movement associated with past pain that produces an anxiety response or the threat of failure at school).
⊃ Self-directed goals encourage self-efficacy and a sense of control.
⊃ Goals allow the therapist, adolescent or parent to assess progress, re-negotiate or withdraw from therapy.
⊃ They create a vision for a positive future where previously there may have been none.
⊃ They help move the adolescent into an 'action' stage of change.
⊃ For some, setting goals is an easily understood process as it suits their personality, social, family or sporting culture. Others ways of describing goals are as 'wants', 'needs', or even 'dreams'. For most adolescents, taking time to express their hopes and dreams for their future is generally an engaging experience in conjunction with strategies to approach the pain.

⭘━ 'Yellow flags'
There are a number of reasons change does not happen, as set out below.
⊃ The adolescent or parent may still believe and fear there is an undiscovered physical cause. – Revisit pain education and, if possible,

suggest a medical case conference to clarify outstanding issues or engage in a graduated exposure exercise.

⊃ They may be on a quest to find out *why* the pain occurs. – As above. Or propose an experiment based on an hypothesis (this is like a graduated exposure exercise). If progress is made, then the hypothesis is likely to be true and the fear lessened (*see* Chapter 2).

⊃ The unchanged behaviour suits both parties at this time, i.e. change threatens; there is a sense of safety for those with unrecognised anxiety (suggest a referral to a psychologist or psychiatrist), or they are awaiting the outcome of a court case for compensation (suggest delaying therapy until after settlement).

Setting goals, and whose are they?

Primarily the goals are the adolescent's, thereby maximising commitment and engagement. However, the parent and therapist may have some suggestions, especially as the adolescent may not identify areas that are less attractive, such as household chores, school attendance or homework. For an adolescent deprived of the pleasurable activities they have formerly taken for granted and on which their self-esteem has been based, nominating these goals may be upsetting to contemplate or may even seem unattainable.

Involving parents

Reasons to include a parent in the process may be:

⊃ to engage the parent in reinforcing or supporting the therapy process

⊃ to support the parent in their role where limits, structure or behavioural boundaries are required

⊃ to get an expanded picture of the adolescent's life, parents are likely to mention issues the adolescent may find anxiety provoking, such as socialising with peers.

Considering that the adolescent is not yet an adult, it is appropriate to include a parent in some way even if the parent is at the same time being encouraged to be less intrusive or enmeshed. Feeling excluded by the therapist may increase a parent's existing separation anxiety. An upset parent may mask this anxiety by becoming critical of the process or the therapist and may withdraw from therapy. Reassure the parent at the first session that they will be kept informed of the content of the sessions, with the agreement of the adolescent. Alternatively, it may be helpful to engage the parent in an individual session where they discuss goals they consider important for their child.

०⊸ 'Yellow flag'

Omitting significant goals

Omitting a significant goal that would normally be expected is usually of more significance than that the adolescent simply forgot to mention it.

⊃ Omitting return to school goal

A classic example is the adolescent or parent not mentioning a goal of returning to school (or work) when there are significant absences from school. Pain can mask many other causes of school or work refusal (this may occur in the form of a request for support for a disability pension). A detailed assessment of the issues for the adolescent and parent is required. Likely issues are separation anxiety, generalised anxiety or specific phobias (such as agoraphobia or social phobia) of the parent or the child. The child may feel responsible for their anxious parent or may be relied on by the parent during the day.

Other *yellow flags* of omission may be:

Not seeking social interaction with peers
➲ This may indicate longstanding problems (e.g. social phobia or Asperger's syndrome) that warrant further assessment by the school or a psychologist.

Not seeking independence in self-care
➲ This may indicate parental enmeshment and delayed or stalled individuation. However, every adolescent and family requires individual assessment within the context of their culture as expectations for independent self-care can be culturally determined.

Case study: Amelia

Amelia was a 15-year-old adolescent who was brought in by both her parents for assessment of her daily leg and whole-body pain. Her pain had started after a fall in gymnastics in her first year of high school. It had gradually increased to the point where she was able to walk only short distances and no longer did gymnastics. Her pain had escalated since her fall so that she had only been able to attend a few hours of school for the last school year. She had maintained her high academic level by completing her schoolwork from home. Her father, who was a teacher at her school, drove her to and from school and arranged for her homework. He was also present at any school discussion involving her management. In confidence the school reported that her parents did not allow her to make independent decisions.

She and her older sister had been competitive in gymnastics; her sister was a high achiever at her school, winning academic and gymnastic prizes as well as being a prefect and sports captain. Amelia's parents were very worried and extremely solicitous of Amelia, encouraging her to stop any activity that caused increase in pain. In the initial assessment the parents answered questions directed to Amelia and when Amelia was specifically requested to answer, she looked to her parents for her answer, finding it difficult to answer independently.

Amelia's medical examination found no underlying pathology causing her persistent pain. Although she was hypermobile and reported daily fatigue, she was not diagnosed as having fibromyalgia. Amelia had become extremely unfit over her years of increasing pain. Amelia and her parents were responsive to explanations provided in an education session on pain physiology and accepted advice on behavioural strategies that would be helpful for Amelia. They expressed relief about finding a clear explanation of what they knew to be their daughter's real pain and a direction for change. It was decided that goal setting should be done with Amelia alone to engage her in her own decision making and to provide her with the experience of successful self-directed action. This session using the Canadian Occupational Performance Measure (usually completed over one hour) took three sessions to complete because Amelia was uncertain of herself, finding great difficulty in deciding for herself – even taking some of her decisions home to discuss with her parents. Her parents had been advised not to make decisions but simply to encourage an independent decision from Amelia and to support her in the execution of her goal. Amelia was taught relaxation and distraction techniques for her pain.

Her goals were discussed at length to ensure that initially goals were short-term ones and that success was guaranteed. Her early success surprised her and gave her great joy and confidence. She was very soon enthusiastic and able to have confidence in making her own longer-term goals (interestingly, these were quite different from her older sister's chosen direction).

Comment

Amelia's early success was dependent on her parents (and Amelia) accepting the explanation for her pain as well as Amelia's underlying personal skills. The change from the family's seeking a cause (why) for the pain, their preparedness to reframe their concept of 'ill' and the learning for Amelia associated with her success in setting her own goals (self-efficacy), made her rapidly independent in self-management of her pain.

Setting goals

A number of issues need to be considered in setting goals.
- Time frame.
- Measurability.
- Number and nature of goals.
- Achievability.

Setting goals that have no time frame

Pros
- less pressure to achieve
- less anxiety making for some
- more flexible – allows for setbacks

Cons
- easily forgotten or lost if not regularly referred to
- goals seem vague or unimportant

Setting goals that have a time frame

Pros
- may be useful if a particular event is anticipated, e.g. school camp, sporting or social event
- support to reach a deadline may help those for whom structure is an aid to motivation

Cons
- may be unachievable within the set time and thus lead to feelings of failure
- inflexible if unexpected events (e.g. pain flare-up, medical intervention, illness) occur, leading to disenchantment with the process of setting goals
- deadline may overrule pacing in order to achieve set timeline, especially in the 'over-doers'

Setting goals where nobody rates or measures success or outcome

Pros
- may seem less threatening initially

Cons
- unclear whether they have been achieved or not
- can cause less motivation in those who enjoy competition or who are not self-motivated

Setting goals where others rate success

Pros
- perceived as more 'objective'
- possibly comparable with others' outcomes

Cons
- rating may not correlate with adolescent's opinion, leading to them feeling the goals are irrelevant
- potential for lack of interest
- potential for anxiety from judgements of others

Setting self-rated goals

Pros
⊃ clear when outcomes are achieved
⊃ aids self-motivation without performance anxiety, especially if re-setting goals is an option
⊃ values the individual's opinion and self-worth
⊃ engages them in considering what details of their goals are important to them

Cons
⊃ can lack objectivity and there is no comparison with others' outcomes

Goals are best if they are:
⊃ based on the client/patient's values
⊃ flexible
⊃ achievable within the foreseeable future
⊃ measurable.

Providing a structure to identify what is important for the adolescent is essential, as there are many areas of activity and behaviour to be considered and it may be overwhelming.

The Canadian Occupational Performance Measure (COPM)

The Canadian Occupational Performance Measure provides a structure that enables discussion of all domains of the adolescent's life – from self-care (personal independence in showering, dressing, community access, mobility, etc.) to the productivity of school, work or play; or leisure that is active (such as sport), passive (such as reading) or social leisure. Goals are rated for 'importance', then five of the most important are chosen to rate for current level of performance and satisfaction with performance. These self-ratings form the basis for the outcome score.

Evidence for the efficacy of the COPM as a tool in outcome measures for pain management is with adult populations.[13,14] Adolescents brainstorm ideas initially to identify those things they *want* to be able to do that they are currently avoiding or are unable to do because of their pain. These may seem to the adolescent to fall in the category of 'dreams' mentioned before. The therapist may enter the dialogue, helping them to find lesser but more achievable goals that, once achieved, will lead to their larger goals. Also, the therapist can refer to the values-based work, suggesting they expand into areas they may not have considered or to include things that they may also *have to* or *need to* do which are unpleasant. An example of a 'need to' sort of goal may be the wearing of a seat belt in a car where the adolescent experiences pain on the chest wall. These goals are likely to be parent or school driven.

Other goals may be around mood- or pain-management behaviours, such as being less grumpy with siblings or not withdrawing to the bedroom when pain flares up. Quantifying frequency and manner of the desired positive behaviour can be difficult but worth the effort. As a way of quantifying change, ask how others will know they have changed, clarify exactly what the new behaviour will look like to others.

Case study: Bernie

(*See* Chapter 10 for more details on Bernie's return to school.)

Doctors had diagnosed Bernie with CRPS in his left knee. Bernie had had a sudden growth spurt in the six months prior to his knee pain and muscle spasms. He was now nearly 6 foot tall, aged 13 years, he used terms like 'weird' to describe his body sensations. He had a history of poor attendance at primary school. Following an initial brief success from a nerve block and an intensive in-patient physiotherapy programme, he had relapsed on return home. He represented for assessment at an outpatient pain-management clinic on crutches and experiencing unmanageable pain and spasms. He had not returned to school following the in-patient stay.

The occupational therapist presented a pain education session, for Bernie and his parents, with particular attention paid to explaining the relationship between anxiety and pain. He was encouraged to associate what particular events or thoughts occurred just prior to flare-ups of pain. He had counselling to help him identify his feelings of anxiety. Bernie required frequent reference to this association throughout his therapy sessions. Following his education session, Bernie, with his mother present, completed the Canadian Occupational Performance Measure identifying the following as his 'wants'.

Self-care:
- To be able to wear long trousers for two hours. (This would allow him to change into shorts at recess or lunch at school if pain continued beyond this time.)
- To walk without crutches for 15 minutes. (This would allow him to walk in the school yard and spend time with friends.)
- To catch the school bus one way at least three times in the week. (His mother who was present identified this goal as a 'want'.)
- To manage spasms independently, wherever they occurred, without needing help from others.
- To initiate sleep within one hour of lights out five nights a week.

Productivity:
- To attend school daily for one month, discounting absences due to illness. (Initially no stipulation for the length of time attended

was made until a return-to-school programme contract had been established.)

- To catch up with school work.
- To spend recess and lunchtimes in the school yard with friends.

Leisure:
Active leisure

- To play basketball in a team. Bernie had enjoyed basketball prior to onset of his CRPS. (This goal was broken down to include lesser goals that were followed up weekly, e.g. two-point jumping, one-point jumping, plus jogging progressing to backyard play with the ball for five minutes, etc.)

Social leisure

- To go out, including to the movies with friends once a month. (He had stopped socialising because of pain and because he was fearful of spasms and shaking.)
- To be able to explain to friends what had happened to him to prevent his attendance at school.

Refining Bernie's goals

Goals were initially 'brainstormed' then refined in discussion to define measurable baselines that enabled Bernie to rate his performance and satisfaction with his performance at a later date and compare the two scores. Goals that were general, such as 'to improve sleep' or 'to go out with friends more' were examined in detail to establish exactly what the problems encountered were, e.g. Bernie had difficulty initiating sleep in less than two hours because he worried. This detail allowed the goal to evolve into 'to initiate sleep within one hour of turning the light off five nights a week' and it directed therapy to focus on strategies to manage anxiety. While 'to play basketball in a team' remained on Bernie's list, it was not chosen as one of the key five that he would rate pre- and post-therapy. It was decided that if he managed 'to run for two minutes non-stop every day', 'to play around with the basketball in the backyard for five minutes three times a week', 'to jump on the spot four jumps a minute for five minutes, four times a week', the achievement of these goals would lead to the ability to play in a team.

The Goal Attainment Scale (GAS)

The Goal Attainment Scale has also been found to be a suitable measure for outcomes in adult chronic pain populations.[15] It provides a structure for individualised goals with a rating for five levels of achievement negotiated between the therapist and the adolescent. Once a goal has been identified, progress can be rated numerically or verbally (which is less negative):

- present level (rated at –2)
- making progress (rated at –1)

⊃   target (short-term goal rated at 0)
⊃   better than expected (rated at +1)
⊃   longer-term or most favourable goal (rated at +2).

A date at which these levels are first nominated is recorded with a projected review date and score. Achieving levels earlier than the review date makes it possible to set a new or modified goal. GAS does not provide a structure that outlines broad areas of the adolescent's life, leaving open the possibility that some areas may be left out. However, it is easily used in conjunction with the Canadian Occupational Performance Measure. It is ideal for use in areas where close monitoring is helpful, such as weekly monitoring of analgesic intake. Both GAS and COPM are flexible, allowing for modification of goals at any time.

Target Complaints

Target Complaints is a client-centred measure originally developed for psychotherapeutic interventions.[16] As the name suggests, the adolescent targets the complaints for which treatment is sought. Since the original paper was published, the method has been standardised in the form of a Target Complaints interview. The method of scoring uses a five-point scale.

Goals can be measured according to:

Number of times . . . x . . . occurs	to get eight hours' sleep five nights a week
% of time . . . x . . .occurs	≥ 50% *reduction* in waking at night from four times per night
length of time for . . . x . . . to occur	that sleep occurs *within the hour*

It is the role of the therapist to help the adolescent make the goals achievable by suggesting limitations or extension to goals, which, if reached, are likely to lead on to the more extended or longer-term goal. It is a significant responsibility to guide this process to something achievable. This is likely to entail close communication with any treating physical therapist or medical practitioner to ensure safety, to prevent unrealistic physical expectations, and to prevent setbacks that come from overdoing activity. Careful pacing is required to achieve success, especially when dealing with the 'over-doers' (Chapter 9 deals with this in more detail).

⊶   'Yellow flags'

The adolescent is unable to identify any goals – this may be a manifestation of depression and the adolescent may require further assessment. It may be that the adolescent or family culture has limited expectations of engagement in life activities, or limited finances.

The therapist may then engage the adolescent and parent in exploring local activities they can manage. Having no goals is a limitation for therapy as there are no drivers for the therapist or the adolescent beyond removing the pain and because boredom leads to focussing on pain.

The adolescent is reluctant to rate their performance or rates their performance as already being high – this alerts the therapist to possible perfectionist characteristics. It may occur when the adolescent finds it intolerable to contemplate a poor performance. Asking a perfectionist to rate their performance is not appropriate; it is best in this circumstance to simply identify areas they would like to improve on. Elaboration of detail is likely to still be possible and helpful. Longer psychological counselling will help deal with perfectionist characteristics. Mindfulness training can assist.

The adolescent is doing everything they want to, need to, or have to do. It may be that they are functioning well in the activities of their choice. This is often so for headache sufferers, who may find themselves able to continue even sporting activities. (*See* Chapter 2 on headaches.) Their goal may simply be to have fewer headaches. (*See* below.)

The only goal is removal of the pain – this expectation needs to be addressed at the very beginning of a therapy programme, perhaps even at the assessment stage. It will be necessary to explain that although a reduction in pain frequency or intensity may occur, nobody can guarantee this. A positive outcome may be that pain is less bothersome. Reference to the physiology of pain information given in Chapter 1 may help, as may repeating the car-driving analogy, i.e. of removing pain from being in the driver's seat, to placing it in the back seat and then into the boot of the car. A good headache diary measuring frequency and intensity of headache is a useful outcome measure and can be a single GAS goal. It is likely to help the adolescent have a sense of efficacy in managing pain if they have regularly practised their chosen strategies, such as relaxation.

References

1 Karoly P, Lecci L. Motivational correlates of self-reported persistent pain in young adults. *Clin J of Pain*. 1997; **13**: 104–9.

2 Miller WR, Rollnick S. *Motivational Interviewing: preparing people to change addictive behaviour.* New York: Guilford Press; 1991.

3 Kerns RD, Habib S. A critical review of the pain readiness to change model. *J Pain*. 2004; **5**(7): 357–67.

4 Strong J, Westbury K, Smith G, *et al*. Treatment outcome in individuals with chronic pain: is the Pain Stages of Change Questionnaire (PSCQ) a useful tool? *Pain*. 2002; **97**: 65–73.

5 Nielson WR, Jensen MP, Kerns RD. Initial development and validation of a Multidimensional Pain Readiness to Change Questionnaire (MPRCQ). *J Pain*. 2003; **104**: 529–37.

6 Glenn B, Burns JW. Pain self-management in the process and outcome of multidisciplinary treatment of chronic pain: evaluation of a stage of change model. *J Behav Med*. 2003; **26**(5): 417–33.

7 McCracken LM, Vowles KE, Eccleston C. Acceptance of chronic pain: component analyses and a revised assessment method. *Pain.* 2000; **107**: 159–66.
8 Greco LA. *ACT for Teens Manual*; 2005. (Available from Laurie Greco, Department of Psychology, University of Missouri – St Louis. Email: grecol@umsl.edu)
9 Hayes S, Strosahl K, editors. *A Practical Guide to Acceptance and Commitment Therapy.* New York: Springer; 2004.
10 Field HA. Motivation-decision model of pain: the role of opioids. In: Flor H, Kalso E, Dostrovsky JO, editors. Proceedings of the 11th World Congress on Pain. Seattle: IASP Press; 2006, pp. 449–59.
11 Miller WR, Zweben Q, DiClemente CC, *et al. Motivational Enhancement Therapy Manual: a clinical research guide for therapists treating individuals with alcohol abuse and dependence* (DHHS Publication No. ADM 92-1894). Washington, DC: US Government Printing Office; 1992.
12 Miller WR, Rollnick S. *Motivational Interviewing: preparing people to change addictive behaviour.* New York: Guilford Press; 1991.
13 Carpenter L, Baker GA, Tyldesley B. The use of the Canadian Occupational Performance Measure as an outcome of a pain management program. *Can J Occ Ther.* 2001; **68**(1): 16–21.
14 Persson E, Rivano-Fischer M, Ekland M. The evaluation of changes in occupational performance among patients in a pain management program. *J Rehab Med.* 2004; **36**(2): 85–91.
15 Azaz C, Stolee P, Prkachin K. The application of goal attainment scaling in chronic pain settings. *J Pain Symp Manag.* 1999; **17**(1): 55–64.
16 Hesbacher P, Rickels K, Weise C. Target symptoms: a promising improvement in psychiatric drug research. *Arch Gen Psychiatry.* 1968; **18**: 595–600.

CHAPTER 6

Dealing with the pain

COPING FACTORS AND MANAGING FLARE-UPS

CHAPTER SUMMARY

This chapter outlines the factors that influence the ability to cope with persistent pain, including health anxiety, fear avoidance, emotional regulation and catastrophising. Passive and active coping strategies are described and discussed with reference to later chapters that will address these in more detail. Key areas of therapy are listed that may constitute an individualised treatment program. This chapter will also discuss the use of attention or distraction and suggest a process for managing acute flare-ups of pain. The reader will need to refer to the later, more detailed accounts of techniques.

Background

There are a number of areas referred to in the literature that influence the adolescent's ability to minimise the disability so frequently associated with persistent pain. Some of these, such as health anxiety and anxiety sensitivity, are closely associated with each other. Others that also influence the adolescent's feelings and behaviours are: emotional regulation, catastrophising, fear avoidance, perceptions of self-efficacy and longstanding coping strategies of avoidance on the part of the adolescent.

Factors that influence coping

Health anxiety

Pain is a survival mechanism, its presence is a threat (of harm). It is designed to interrupt our concentration and to demand attention over what may be multiple other demands on our attention. It is normal to be vigilant to pain. The degree of vigilance changes according to a number of factors.

We are likely to attend more to a pain (i.e. be more vigilant), if it has a *high degree* of threat (e.g. likelihood of disability), if it is an *unusually intense* pain, or if its *cause or meaning is unpredictable*. Once pain occurs we appraise the degree of threat. If we appraise the threat as not high or if we understand why it is there, we are likely to continue with our activity or rest appropriately until healing occurs. The pain may continue to interrupt our concentration on tasks but as there is no significant threat, there is no anxiety associated with the presence of the pain. The pain is likely to be predictable and possibly time limited. This cycle is different for the adolescent seeking help for the management of pain. The nature of chronic or persistent pain is that it is not apparently time limited. In this case, the pain may be unpredictable, perceived as disabling and mysterious. The degree of vigilance increases to become hypervigilance.

Hypervigilance is normal vigilance in the abnormal situation of the presence of persistent or chronic pain. Once a threat (of disability or harm) is perceived, there is difficulty in disengaging from the threatening signal, i.e. the pain, thereby fuelling the hypervigilance cycle.

Hypervigilance to pain and other somatic sensations is associated with catastrophic thoughts (appraisals of threat) and more reporting of symptoms. Beliefs or thoughts that pain equates to harm or damage, that activity should be avoided or that pain is a mystery are associated with poor outcomes. The individual may develop avoidant behavioural responses (avoidance of movement, situations or thoughts associated with threat).

Hypervigilance and negative appraisals of body sensations are associated with a number of areas in the research literature. Treatments directly targeting the threat value of pain are likely to be more effective than attempts to distract from, remove or modify the thought of threat.[1,2,3] Treatment involves graduated exposure to the threat (movement, anxious thoughts, negative body sensations, etc).

Anxiety sensitivity

Anxiety sensitivity refers to the fear of anxiety-related sensations that are interpreted as having potentially harmful somatic, psychological or social consequences. Examples may be a fear of blushing and public embarrassment or a fear of a thumping heart that could be a heart attack, these fears being associated with anxiety states and phobias. Studies in adults with chronic pain, who are negatively affected by their pain experiences, have shown higher anxiety sensitivity and pain-related anxiety.[4] It is hypothesised that people with persistent pain are prone to develop fear of pain and that high levels of somatisation and panic-like symptoms alter their perception of bodily sensation. This can lead to catastrophic interpretations of the cause of the pain leading to a fear of the sensations.

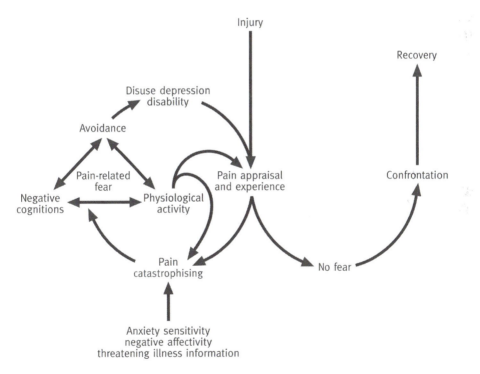

FIGURE 6.1 Amended Vlayen-Linton fear-avoidance model of chronic pain

Reproduced with the permission of the Association for Behavioral and Cognitive Therapies. Norton PJ, Asmundson GJG. Amending the fear-avoidance model of chronic pain: what is the role for physiological arousal? *Behav Ther.* 2003; **34**: 19.

In the healthy adolescent population, anxiety sensitivity is significantly related to pain anxiety symptoms and an increase in reported experience of pain.[5]

Treatment is designed to provide new experiences and appraisals that extinguish the avoidant behaviours. Graduated exposure to movement, activity and exercise (*see* Chapter 9) accompanied by breathing techniques and mindfulness (*see* Chapter 7) provides new coping experiences.

Fear avoidance

Fear avoidance in the adult pain population is a predictor of disability.[6] Clinically it is observable in some adolescents with persistent pain. Fear avoidance involves the expectation of consequences of certain actions on pain. 'If I move too much/that way/too fast, etc., it will hurt' (i.e. there is the expectation of pain, a perception of threat leading to hypervigilance, resulting in avoidance of movement and guarding behaviours). Mindful observance of thoughts and graduated exposure to movement, activity and exercise is designed to extinguish the avoidant behaviours.

Emotional regulation[7]

Emotional regulation is defined as the ability to redirect, control and modify emotionally arousing situations and is associated with both internalising and externalising problems.[8] Adolescents with persistent pain have higher incidence than the normal population.[9] Impoverished emotional awareness, poor emotional understanding, and dysregulated emotional expression are associated with internalising disorders such as anxiety and depression.[10,11]

Emotional regulation impacts on how we are 'affected' by an event. The emotional development of an individual is dependent on the level of responsiveness and attunement of the mother to the child. A mother who is highly sensitive to her child's distress or emotional cues will help to maintain the optimum level of arousal. This, in turn, will influence her child's ability to regulate their emotions in terms of intensity, sensitivity, tolerance, expression and repression. Increasing levels of maternal emotional distress are associated with child somatisation, anxiety, depression and reduced physical function.[12]

⟲ 'Yellow flags'

⟳ If an adolescent continually responds to emotionally provocative events with a 'poker face' or otherwise unresponsive behaviour, this could be a source of concern, given that the expression of negative emotions in constructive ways is deemed to be adaptive.

⟳ It may be of concern if an adolescent is unable to recognise the physiological sensations in their body that accompany particular emotions such as fear or anger. A difficulty may become apparent in the education process (*see* Chapter 1), during discussion about thoughts and feelings influencing pain.

⟳ An adolescent who overreacts (e.g. tears of frustration or extreme facial expression of dislike) to minor precipitants such as an unwanted change, suggestions of new ideas, discomforts or the prospect of effort (such as getting out of bed early) can cause those around them – parents (and themselves) to avoid these minor precipitants. This cushions them from appropriate learning experiences that would otherwise increase their tolerance and ability to appropriately regulate their emotions.

↻ If a child's emotional style is overly emotional in reaction to minor precipitants or is minimally responsive or responds in a way that is incongruent with the situation, then the child's emotional style may impede their ability to initiate or maintain friendships.

It may be that the child needs help with decoding others' emotions or understanding the causes and consequences of emotional responses. Social skills training with an emphasis on emotional regulation skills may be appropriate with the assistance of a psychologist. Chapter 3 deals with this further, in the context of the family environment.

Catastrophising

Catastrophising is expecting or worrying about major negative consequences from a situation or event. This may be regarded as a heightened interpretation of threat leading to hypervigilance. An event of minor importance is associated with a greater experience of pain and dysfunction. Thoughts such as 'I can't stand it anymore', 'I can't go on', 'I feel I have red hot pokers in my head', 'I think I have a tumour no one has found', 'I worry whether it will end' characterise catastrophising. Catastrophising language (in adults with chronic pain) is associated with changes in the cerebral cortex and an increase in the experience of pain and lower psychosocial and physical functioning.[13,14] In adolescents with chronic pain, catastrophising accounts for pain, disability and somatic complaints and is the best predictor of emotional distress in those adolescents with high levels of depression, disability and anxiety.[15] Catastrophising is understood in the context of communicating distress to significant others, i.e. seeking emotional support to cope with the pain.[16]

A thought diary and mindfulness training teaches an attitude of detached observation of catastrophising and other unhelpful language (*see* Chapters 7 and 8).

'What do I do with the pain when it comes?'

This is the question uppermost in the mind of the adolescent and family, or alternatively, 'What can *you* do to help me . . .' The unspoken end of the question is '. . . *to make it go away*'. Making the pain go away is frequently the overt agenda for the adolescent and family seeking help (sometimes this agenda is covert and needs to be made overt). Changing that agenda is the first step in a pain program. Pain coping strategies are not directed at lessening or removing pain; they are directed at achieving a healthy, fulfilling lifestyle, and at the pain being less of a bother or a worry in the context of the individual's life. In the process, the pain may indirectly also be reduced.

Passive and active coping

Maladaptive coping associated with poorer outcomes may be either of the following.

➲ Avoidance (sometimes referred to as avoidant coping) with habitual withdrawal when pain (or other unpleasant events or emotions) occurs, leading to increasing social isolation and focus on pain. The adolescent may be also avoiding anxiety associated with unpleasant social situations such as bullying.

➲ Hoping and praying thoughts such as 'I cope by just hoping it will go away'. This often results in waiting and resting until it goes.

Adaptive strategies associated with less pain and better function include the following.

➲ Observing automatic thoughts and recognising whether they are helpful or not. 'There it is again, it's only pain not damage' and choosing to keep going despite the pain.

➲ Pacing activity to maintain exercise over time – despite the pain (*see* Chapter 9).

➲ Using relaxation/breathing/mindfulness exercises (*see* Chapter 7).

➲ Persisting with tasks, sometimes called 'approach' coping, is the opposite of avoidance. Persisting with tasks (*see* Chapters 5 and 7) regardless of pain provides new learning that reinforces new, functional behaviour patterns. These new experiences change the adolescent's belief in their ability to be effective in the face of pain.

Self-efficacy

A belief in one's ability to take action when in pain, described by Bandura as self-efficacy, increases pain tolerance in laboratory conditions.[17] It is self-evident that adolescents presenting for help in managing pain do not believe in their ability to manage or cope. One can speculate, perhaps, that in non-laboratory conditions, this would also translate to longer times of tolerance to pain. Skills training (mindfulness, breathing techniques, helpful language, task persistence, pacing and problem solving) directs the actions which may contribute to self-efficacy and the belief in one's ability to cope despite the pain[18] (*see* Chapters 5, 7, 8 and 9).

It would seem that self-efficacy is also a concept related to coping strategies in that the strategies employed are the vehicle for the belief.

Table 6.1 is a summary of signs likely to negatively influence disability and actions a therapist may use to positively influence abilities.

TABLE 6.1 Summary of signs

POOR COPERS	THERAPIST ACTION
Don't believe they can do anything about the pain or their situation (they feel 'stuck', hopeless or a victim)	Teach skills – use diary to record and reinforce action (pacing, breathing, thought awareness, etc.). Set short, achievable, value-based goals
Others take action on their behalf, or attempt to relieve the pain, e.g. masseurs (parental action may deprive them of coping experiences)	Assist significant 'others' to understand that the adolescent needs to learn independent experiences of coping with discomfort and pain
Internalise or avoid negative emotions/sensations – social withdrawal. Unable to ask for help with problems.	Mindfulness of acceptance and exposure to negative events. (Record progress in diary.) Facilitate expression of same at school, at home or in therapy. Set up networks of support
Focus on the pain	Engage the adolescent in meaningful activity and teach acceptance of interruptive nature of pain – teach the ability to refocus – sensate training
Inability to or difficulty in recognising their feelings	Use diary to recognise associations of events/thoughts/emotions/pain
Inability to or difficulty in regulating their emotions and sensations	Assist in recognising the thought that accompanies the feeling (*see* Chapter 6)
Modelling pain behaviour in the family	Detached observation of language (catastrophising, etc.), breathing techniques and commitment to values-based action. Social skills training
	Values-based work in specific domains to identify positive models in their environment. Role-play pain behaviour and discuss consequences

Pain: to attend or distract?

Distraction is the purposeful focussing of the mind on an alternative subject from that which is unpleasant, e.g. a worrying thought or sensation, pain. It may be an effective method of coping with acute pain, as shown in experimental studies with children and adolescents.[19] However, it is unlikely to be a successful strategy for an adolescent whose habitual coping habits are avoidant. Attempting to control the pain by using distraction to avoid it only increases the threat (and the hypervigilance) associated with the feared object (pain). The role of hypervigilance and attention to pain and other negative somatic sensations has been noted previously. Literature that focuses on adults adjusting to chronic pain show mixed results for the use of distraction in coping with pain in experimental circumstances.[20] Furthermore, distraction from pain in adults with chronic pain during a pain-inducing task is associated with greater post-activity pain and no change in reported pain during the task.[21]

Distraction may have some useful role in circumstances where it is not accompanied by avoidant behaviour, i.e. as a means of persevering with an activity that is engaging, valuable and rewarding to the adolescent. Where this is possible, the interruptive nature of pain is accepted by the adolescent and they are not attempting to *not have* the pain. Engaging in competing engrossments are pain-management tools (*see* Chapter 5 (discussion of values-based goals) or 'Imagery and visualisation' in Chapter 7) as attentional resources available at any given moment are severely limited.[22]

The degree of difficulty of the distraction task does not appear to be significant. However, distraction with emotional content is likely to be significant in altering pain perception, i.e. distraction associated with pleasant cognitions or images produce a significant increase in pain tolerance compared with anger-based cognitions.[23]

Case study of Maria

Maria was a 15-year-old adolescent with congenital limb deficiency who wore prostheses on each lower limb. Maria had complex peer and family problems as well as debilitating pain in her stumps. At presentation she was unable to endure wearing her prostheses. She described herself as stubborn, refusing to use a wheelchair. She was demanding of her mother. Despite one of her values being to be independent, she relied on her mother to drive her wherever she wanted to go. She was prone to emotional outbursts at home when either her mother, her mother's partner or her brother crossed her. She displayed the same emotional response in sessions when subjects she did not want to address were raised, e.g. she would shout or cry when suggestions for pacing herself using either crutches or wheelchair were made. Also, despite the stated value she placed on higher education, she was not attending school. She stated that this was because she could not tolerate her peers.

With family therapy and counselling regarding emotional regulation, Maria's relationships with her separated parents, her mother's partner and her brother improved. She learned to accept the presence of her pain while pursuing her goals. She increased her prosthesis usage and was able to attend school in the manner she wanted. She learned to be more tolerant of her peers and made some friends. Maria used the image of a mermaid when pain flared in her stumps, especially while catching the bus home from school. This allowed her to feel consistent with her value-based goal of independence.

Comment

The initial strategies used by Maria were avoidant, i.e. social withdrawal, avoidance of circumstances that caused unpleasant feelings such as using her wheelchair. Maria learned to modify her reaction to her emotions and to face and accept her unpleasant feelings, so that she was able to use imagery in a way that was not avoidant.

Summary of key areas of therapy

Individualise a program for each adolescent and family based on combinations of the following.

- **Assess objects or circumstances of avoidance** and patterns of behaviour (this may include areas other than pain, such as unwanted emotions like frustration, sensitivity to anxiety; or unpleasant social circumstances like bullying, fear of academic failure, etc.).

- **Assess patterns of pain** and address likely causes if possible. If pain is worse later in the day, pace activity so that there is less at the beginning of the day and/or implement relaxation earlier in the day *before* pain increases. If relaxation or breathing techniques are useful as a means of quietening the nervous system, make sure relaxation is initially practised and learned at times when pain is not particularly magnified so that when pain does increase, the adolescent already has the skills to apply. Make sure that the coping appraisals are positive (*see* Chapter 8).

- **Identify values-based activities** or tasks that are likely to be difficult to persist with when pain interrupts; use these as the basis for programme that gradually exposes the adolescent to restricted activities and increasing task persistence. Set baselines of endurance if appropriate (*see* Chapters 5 and 9).

- **Educate** on pain physiology, body function, medical condition and psychological processes, tailoring content and emphasis to address the individual's needs.

- **Problem-solve with school** about likely causes of stress (school culture regarding pain, general academic performance, particular subjects or teachers or school-yard behaviour etc. (*see* Chapter 10). Assist in setting up local support networks for ongoing problem solving and support.

- **Utilise what already works** for the adolescent in task persistence (taking into account any avoidant behaviours).

- **Teach a new skill early** in therapy and implement a means by which this can be practised at home/school early in therapy. Breathing awareness and thought awareness or relaxation in the first session gives the adolescent something to act with immediately – recording home-based practice invites commitment to the next session. Encourage practising in various applied circumstances.

- **Use a diary** to record and reinforce new behaviours (not to record pain).

- **Identify what subject or image has positive emotional content** if using distraction for specific tasks for that adolescent. (The subject may be anything from being a mermaid, to making a pizza to milking a cow!) Talk them through a visualisation of this image (*see* Case study of Maria).

- **Have agreed activities** that the adolescent identifies as very valued and engrossing – computer games, talking to friends on the phone, playing with their pet. Prepare them for the likelihood of pain interrupting their activity (discuss acceptance of their pain). Success lies in *their ability to reapply attention* and task persistence after pain has interrupted. The engagement in a task is not designed or expected to remove or diminish pain, though they may find they forget about it if engrossed in meaningful activity.

➲ **Teach applied relaxation and mindfulness** skills and how they can be applied in situ. Talk through what will work for them. After the initial skill has been learned, it is imperative to *apply* relaxation or mindfulness when walking, writing, at the shops or in class with the eyes open (*see* Chapter 7).

➲ **Coaching in mindfulness: observe, breathe, and allow** negative thoughts or sensations. It is helpful to be able to be aware of thoughts and query whether they are helpful. 'That old story again!'

➲ *Gradually* **expose the adolescent to situations they find difficult** and apply the skills already taught (mindfulness, breathing, etc.). These may be physical, social or psychological difficulties such as being still, tolerating loud noises, sitting, being in the classroom or school yard or feeling anxious when away from their mother. Acknowledge the increase in tolerance levels and ability to persist with the task.

➲ **Add individualised flash cards** that assist in recognising unpleasant or unhelpful thoughts (*see* Chapter 8).

➲ **Make a flare-up plan** (see below).

➲ **Follow up home/school practice *within a week*.** Waiting for several weeks for a follow-up session can be troublesome. An accumulation of negative experiences or problems that arise can reinforce old experiences, past learning and interpretations of failure. These can overwhelm any new, more fragile perceptions of success which need to be reinforced immediately.

➲ **Positively reinforce any success.** Ask the adolescent to look for their own signs of success in the first few weeks. Look at the consequences of their changed behaviour (*see* 'Using a diary' in Chapter 8). These experiences become cumulative and more believable as the adolescent gradually extinguishes old behaviours. Success may initially simply be the ability to take an action – the ability to persevere in the face of pain and the commitment to continue the practice without the reward of immediate pain relief. Reinforcement may be the recording of the increasing number of times action was taken by the adolescent or the decrease in pain behaviour as observed by others (talking about pain or withdrawing).

Any of these strategies can be formulated into a goal (*see* Chapter 5). Suggest the adolescent choose a reward for themselves for self-rated success. Parents may need to be part of this process as the reward may involve their time (or money!). Some determined adolescents are even able to deprive themselves of a particular pleasure and to use the reinstatement of that pleasure as a reward! e.g. 'I won't have another massage until I am able to walk round the block.'

Managing an acute pain flare-up

Discuss with the adolescent and parents the pain patterns and coping strategies identified in the initial assessment (e.g. avoidance behaviours including withdrawal from activities, crying, massage, talking to mother, etc.). Query whether they are effective in reducing pain. If the answer is 'No' then discuss with them whether they are leading the life they want to lead.

If avoidance behaviours are strongly represented it is likely that the adolescent will not attend therapy when a flare-up occurs. It is important to address the expectation of attendance at appointments at the time of a flare-up. An attitude of willingness is required for change so that if pain flares up, there is a willingness to commit to therapy despite pain. A pain flare-up is a most important and helpful time to attend a session as the therapist will actively coach the adolescent through the pain flare-up. Attending a session despite pain is the first act of commitment and perseverance.

Before a flare-up occurs or as soon as possible in therapy:
⊃ clarify the agenda implicit in the language of *managing a flare-up* (i.e. expectation of the ability to continue activity *despite* pain as opposed to the removal of pain)
⊃ teach and practise breathing and mindfulness techniques early on and when pain has not flared up (*see* Chapter 7)
⊃ work with the adolescent on the following questions, with the adolescent providing answers (record the answers in a diary or use them to create flash-cards as future reminders – *see* Chapter 8 and Handout 12 in the Appendix)

Examples:

WHAT DO I KNOW ABOUT A PAIN FLARE-UP?	WHAT CAN I DO WHEN PAIN FLARES?
Flare-ups are unpredictable	I can use my breathing techniques
They come and they go away	I can continue with my activities even if pain interrupts sometimes
They are only pain, not harm	
I can't predict how long they will last	I can pace myself to keep going
	I can act differently from my negative thoughts/emotions
	I can mind how I think – I can use my flash cards
	I can keep going and choose my own direction

⊃ Make sure the family is prepared and knows helpful behaviour patterns (*see* Chapter 3)
⊃ Have an agreed plan that includes:

- everyone's behaviours at the time, i.e. what others will do (*see* Handout 4: Managing pain behaviours in the Appendix) and what the adolescent will do (use diary, mindfulness, breathing techniques, flashcards, pacing, etc.)
- chosen activities to engage focus, e.g. talking on the phone to friends, re-engaging with current task (*see* 'Mindfulness of a task' in Chapter 7)
- a follow-up session close to the event to acknowledge positive actions taken.

Case study: Megan

Megan was a 16-year-old girl who had loved her school netball and described herself as 'sporty'. She had a vocational goal of teaching physical education. Prior to her pain, she had been an 'A' student, and had enjoyed her art and her social life. She presented at the pain management clinic with a history of bilateral foot pain and lower leg pain lasting for two years. Functionally she was unable to stand or walk for longer than 15 minutes without significantly increasing her pain and was unable to sit cross-legged on the floor. Her pain increased during the day so that her concentration in the late afternoon was reduced to 15 minutes in class. She was missing two or three days of school per week because of pain and fatigue due to sleep problems. She reported significant mood change, from being a happy popular girl to a sad withdrawn person.

She first noticed pain after sport, two years ago. Initially, this pain lasted for three weeks. She visited her GP, and had an X-ray which showed nothing unusual. After one year of intermittent but increasing pain, Megan was having difficulty walking without unmanageable pain, her calves became stiff, she found sleep difficult to initiate and maintain, and she was forced to stop all sport. Her mother described a considerable decline in mood over this time. A sports medicine doctor treated her with ultrasound and taped her ankles and she was issued with orthotics. She was diagnosed with plantar fasciitis by a physiotherapist and new orthotics were issued. She was again treated with ultrasound and acupuncture but with no substantial relief. In the second year she was referred to an orthopaedic surgeon who ordered a CAT scan and referred her to the pain-management clinic.

Following assessment and an education session, Megan identified her goals as wanting to play one quarter of netball, to increase her ability to concentrate despite pain, to learn to initiate sleep earlier and to establish regular morning rising patterns to enable timely attendance at school. Her final goal was to not refuse social engagements because of pain.

Megan's education session focussed on the 'pain gate' (*see*

Chapter 1) and the physiological basis for non-pharmacological pain-management strategies of relaxation, distraction and pacing. Initially her mother described feeling hopeless and ineffective. Following the education session she described a sense of relief, as she envisaged some direction for Megan to self-manage and her role as support in this process. She felt she understood why, despite her best efforts, she was not able to alter her daughter's pain.

Megan learned to identify for herself a number of underlying thoughts that were likely to be upsetting and unhelpful. She was aware that she repeatedly said that if she could only find out 'why' she had the pain then everything would be all right. Also, she identified that she felt angry, saying to herself that it was 'unfair'. She also felt unhappy about herself, feeling fat and lazy since she was not playing sport anymore. At times she resorted to punching her calves from loathing and anger. She worried about her future as a teacher if she was unable to walk or stand.

In the next session Megan was taught mindfulness meditation. She also learned relaxation lying prone on the floor and was taught to use meditation in her daily life (walking, in class, etc.). Megan undertook to practise this once a day before bedtime and the applied version a minimum of three times a day for the next week. In particular, she was to practise when she did not have an increase in pain as well as when she noticed any discomfort. She was to use a record sheet to assist her in remembering her practice (*see* Handout 11 in the Appendix).

In the session the following week, practical difficulties around her meditation were sorted out. Megan had to be reminded not to expect instant change and that this was just a process of training the body – just as she had done in sport.

In the first weeks of attendance at the pain-management clinic, her treating orthopaedic surgeon identified, from the results of the CAT scan, that Megan had congenital fused bones in both feet.

Following an orthopaedic case conference it was agreed that an operation would be of dubious benefit. This was a clarifying process for the family and enabled greater acceptance of the ongoing nature of the pain and its non-pharmacological management. The family decided not to pursue any further medical intervention.

Prior to achieving this clarity regarding her medical status, the possible outcomes had already been discussed:
a. medical intervention that may remove pain
b. medical intervention that does not remove pain
c. the existing status quo.

The family had partially accepted the likelihood of ongoing pain and the non-medical management. The resolution of the CAT scan removed the constant 'Why?' and enabled them to take action. Megan began an intense physiotherapy programme aimed at stretching her calf muscles and hamstrings and to assist with her plantar fascia pain.

Megan used a homework diary to record her thoughts when she felt angry, sad, worried or in pain. These were brought to one session to work on identifying triggers and recurring unhelpful thoughts. She constructed on her computer a series of flash-cards that she kept in her diary at school and on her bedroom wall. These helped her recognise her 'old story' thoughts at short notice.

Megan worked on identifying her values. She found that she could satisfy her values to feel positive and enjoy her body in practising yoga. She changed her original goal from netball to applying for an art scholarship. She came to see herself as directed to her skills in art rather than her sport as a vocation. She accepted that she had 'matured' from a sport phase and she need not depend on this as her primary source of social life.

With her approval, her school was contacted regarding her diagnosis and the necessity for Megan to modify aspects of her hospitality and life drawing classes and alternatives to using multiple stairs. One letter was written for dissemination to all her teachers while a second letter requested special consideration during exam times to allow her to withdraw if required to practise meditation.

Megan continued to have days of pain flare-up when she was required to limit her walking; however, she ceased to think that this was unfair as she was increasingly rewarded in her new directions, devoting more time to art. Working out a process to pace herself at social events was aimed at ensuring her continuing participation. By her fourth session she had successfully managed her pain at one social event. She learned to recognise the preliminary signs of a flare-up and would immediately practise her meditation, wherever she was. She learned to take action early, recognising that hoping that a flare-up would not occur was not a helpful thought. She was able to say with belief to herself that she could continue despite a flare-up and that it would pass. In this way she felt that her flare-ups were less frequent and less significant in her life.

Megan's sleep also improved with her use of relaxation/meditation and reduction of her worries about her future and her school problems. She eventually won a scholarship to an art college managing the considerable stress involved in the application and examination process.

Case study: Hannah
(*See* Chapter 8 for a more elaborated background to this case.)

Hannah was a 15-year-old high school student whose vocational dream was to serve in the army. During cadet training she had been sexually abused by one of her superiors. Subsequently, she had steadfastly refused all counselling. Hannah had an unswerving commitment to the army as a career. Hannah had injured her shoulder at the time of the traumatic incident.

Despite intensive physical rehabilitation on her shoulder, she maintained a dysfunctional, guarded posture of the arm which led to increasing stiffness and pain. Just as she endured and pushed through the abuse, she continued to attempt to push through pain.

Hannah initially described her most useful pain coping strategy as distraction and ignoring pain. In the course of a longer than usual rehabilitation programme it was this strategy that was found to be contributing most to her lack of progress.

Hannah's characteristic coping was inflexible and avoidant; she ignored her feelings in order to push through pain. This avoidance and pushing was probably an established mindset (even prior to her abuse event) given her long-established passion for the military. It was a mindset that did not help her deal with her trauma either. Hannah's ineffective use of distraction had set up a vicious cycle of overdoing activity, increase in pain and increase in fear/avoidance of activity – all of which she continued to avoid recognising. Hannah's arm function had decreased over time despite using distraction. For her, cognitive distraction activities became a form of avoidance. When Hannah stopped distracting from her pain and 'looked the fear in the face' in mindfulness meditation, she was able to make physical progress. She began to find the pain more acceptable, less fearful and was able to persist with her rehabilitation exercises.

References

1 Eccleston C, Crombez G. Pain demands attention: a cognitive-affective model of the interruptive function of pain. *Psychol Bull.* 1999; **125**: 356–66.
2 Van Damme S, Crombez G, Eccleston C, *et al.* The role of hypervigilance in the experience of pain. In: Asmundson GJG, Vlaeyen JWS, Crombez G, editors. *Understanding and Treating Fear of Pain.* Oxford: OUP, pp. 71–90.
3 Aldrich S, Eccleston C, Crombez G. Worrying about chronic pain: vigilance to threat and misdirected problem solving. *Behav Res Ther.* 2000; **38**: 457–70.
4 Asmundson GJG, Norton GR. Anxiety sensitivity in patients with physically unexplained chronic back pain: a preliminary report. *Beh Res and Ther.* 1995; **33**: 771–7.
5 Muris P, Vlaeyen J, Meesters C. The relationship between anxiety, sensitivity and fear of pain in healthy adolescents. *Beh Res and Ther.* 2001; **39**(11): 1357–68.
6 Asmundson GJG, Norton PJ, Norton GR. Beyond pain: the role of fear and avoidance in chronicity. *Clin Psych Rev.* 1999; **19**: 97–119.
7 Zeman J, Cassano M, Perry-Parrish C, *et al.* Emotion regulation in children and adolescents. *J Dev Behav Pediatr.* 2006; **27**(2): 155–68.

8 Eisenberg N, Cumberland AJ, Spinran TL, *et al*. The relations of regulation and emotionality to children's externalising and internalising problem behaviour. *Child Dev*. 2001; **72**: 1112–34.

9 Burba B, Oswald R, Grigaliunien V, *et al*. A controlled study of alexithymia in adolescent patients with persistent somatoform pain disorder. *Can J Psychiat*. 2006; **51**(7): 468–71.

10 Southam-Gerow MA, Kendall PC. Emotion regulation and understanding: implications for child psychopathology and therapy. *Clin Psychol Rev*. 2002; **22**: 189–222.

11 Suveg C, Zeman J. Emotion regulation in anxiety-disordered children. *J Clin Child Adolesc Psychol*. 2004; **33**: 750–9.

12 Franks S, Joyce M, Chalkiadis G. Maternal and child emotional regulation in paediatric chronic pain. In: Flor H, Kalso E, Dostrovsky JO, editors. *Proceedings of the 11th World Congress on Pain*; Seattle: IASP Press; 2006, pp. 597–606.

13 Knost B, Flor H, Braun C, *et al*. Cerebral processing of words and the development of chronic pain. *Psychophysiol*. 1997; **34**(4): 474–81.

14 Turner JA, Jensen MP, Romano JM. Do beliefs, coping and catastrophising independently predict functioning in patients with chronic pain? *Pain*. 2000; **85**: 115–25.

15 Vervoort T, Goubert L, Eccleston C, *et al*. Catastrophic thinking about pain is independently associated with pain severity, disability and somatic complaints in school children and children with chronic pain. *J Pediatr Psychol*. 2006; **31**(7): 674–83.

16 Eccleston C, Crombez G, Scotford A, *et al*. Adolescent chronic pain: patterns and predictors of emotional distress in adolescents with chronic pain and their parents. *Pain*. 2004; **108**(3): 221–9.

17 Bandura A, O'Leary A, Barr Taylor C, *et al*. Perceived self-efficacy and pain control: opioid and non-opioid mechanisms. *J Person and Soc Psychol*. 1987; **53**(3): 563–71.

18 Bursch B, Tsao J, Meldrum M, *et al*. Preliminary validation of a self-efficacy scale for child functioning despite chronic pain (child and parent versions). *Pain*. 2006; **125**: 35–42.

19 Reid G, Gilbert C, McGrath P. The Pain Coping Questionnaire: preliminary validation. *Pain*. 1998; **76**(1–2): 83–96.

20 Jensen MT, Karoly P. Control beliefs, coping efforts and adjustment to chronic pain. *J Consul Clin Psychol*. 1991; **59**: 431–8.

21 Goubert L, Crombez G, Eccleston C, *et al*. Distraction from chronic pain during a pain-inducing activity is associated with greater post-activity pain. *Pain*. 2004; **110**(1–2): 220–7.

22 Kahneman D. *Attention and Effort*. Englewood Cliffs NJ: Prentice Hall; 1973.

23 Stevens MJ, Heise RR, Pfost KS. Consumption of attention versus affect elicited by cognitions in modifying acute pain. *Psychol Rep*. 1998; **64**(1): 284–6.

CHAPTER 7

Mindfulness, relaxation and imagery

HOW TO TEACH SKILLS TO THE ADOLESCENT

CHAPTER SUMMARY

This chapter presents a brief history of relaxation and discusses definition, treatment and limitations on evidence in this area. Basic principles that underpin teaching skills and the barriers that a therapist may meet are addressed. Scripts for teaching breathing awareness, mindfulness exercises and the use of imagery are elaborated. A sheet for recording practice is given.

Background

Research in this area is dogged by a lack of clarity of definitions and standardised training for practices of relaxation, mediation, mindfulness, and visualisation. Good evidence exists for the effectiveness of relaxation in reducing the severity and frequency of chronic headache in children and adolescents.[1] There is a paucity of research in conditions other than headache. Although there is a lack of agreed shared practices and definitions, this is not proof positive that particular techniques practised by a particular therapist are without merit. Some version of relaxation, meditation, or visualisation is usually found by practitioners to be useful in the process of managing a life with persistent pain. Some studies of adults with chronic pain have shown that practising of relaxation produces a sense of calm and that the regular practice of mindfulness meditation resulted in reduction of present-moment pain and a reduction in other negative symptomatology associated with pain.[2] There is a myriad of descriptions, formats and theories in this area. In analysing the elements of relaxation and its various forms and their outcome, a simple maxim is that 'you get what you practise'.[3] This chapter aims to present a broad picture of some common practices.

There are a number of methods that have been studied since the father of relaxation (Jacobson) developed progressive relaxation using a muscular tense-release technique in 1929. He postulated that quietening muscle activity also quietened proprioceptive input and that this, in turn, quieted autonomic and cortical arousal. Later research on animals verified that posterior hypothalamic and sympathetic arousal is directly related to muscular proprioceptive activity.

The behaviourist Joseph Wolpe used an adapted method of progressive relaxation for behavioural therapy for sympathetic states of anxiety. Herbert Benson also presented a parasympathetic theory of relaxation using secular meditation. He proposed that all training procedures comprise the same basic ingredients. Other investigators have applied a 'cognitive'/'somatic' distinction to types of relaxation. Somatic relaxation involves muscular, visceral or neurological mechanisms induced by progressive relaxation technique, EMG biofeedback and physical exercise. Cognitive relaxation consists of the subjective experience of calm, induced by meditation, hypnosis and imagery methods.

Measures of relaxed behaviour can be described as *overt* and/or *covert*. *Overt* is that which is observable by the audience or trainer while *covert* is only experienced or observed by the subject or trainee. An example of overtly relaxed behaviour is a relaxed posture, eyes closed and still, steady regular breathing, while covert relaxed behaviour may be a felt as slower heart beat, a feeling of heaviness in the muscles, or a feeling of calmness in the mind. Covert behaviour is only measurable by self-report of the adolescent observing or attending to interactional, silent or verbal use of imagery – 'seeing in the absence of the thing seen'. Making movies with the mind or using the 'mind's eye' are other ways of describing this process.

The classic unrelaxed visceral behaviour involving the autonomic nervous system and the release of adrenalin is the 'fight-or-flight' response particular to the individual. Some people respond by sweating or flushing, others by blanching or even fainting. Some may experience bowel discomfort and a sudden need to use the toilet. In the release of adrenalin in the 'fight-or-flight' response, most people experience an increase in heart and breathing rate, muscle tension generally, or perhaps in particular places. These may be in the stomach, jaw, neck or shoulders, and this is sometimes accompanied by other unpleasant sensations such as nausea or tension-type headaches or dizziness.

Treatment

In pain management, the aim of any of the practices described is to allow sustained function in life. Therefore, best practices are those that are portable, useable in many situations and that do not require special equipment, environments or other persons (i.e. do not require special background music, aromas or even complete silence). Personal experience of different forms of relaxation/meditation, etc. and reflection upon that experience are likely to be helpful for the therapist's teaching and will encourage confidence and creativity. It is an asset for a therapist to be able to offer alternative forms as required. Taped scripts may, for instance become over-familiar and predictable over time. If using one of these, suggest that the adolescent should take breaks from the tape and create their own 'internal' script independently. Alternatively, using a range of tapes may provide sufficient interest. Teach the adolescent that it is their responsibility to keep the process enduring over time. Similarly, understanding the difficulties that arise in establishing a routine of daily practice is also helpful for the therapist and helps them problem-solve for the adolescent.

Basic principles for teaching skills

Some of the following suggestions are targeted at particular needs, and clinicians will need to choose what is most appropriate to spend time on. The need will depend on the adolescent's anxiety, co-operation or interest level, and which technique is the focus, i.e. mindfulness, diaphragm breathing or relaxation.

Educate about the fundamentals of breathing. To explain the mechanics it can be useful to draw a picture of how the diaphragm is attached to the lungs and how, when it contracts, it presses down into the abdominal cavity causing increased pressure and the area around the navel to be pressed out like a balloon. This area sinks back down as the contraction relaxes or 'lets go'. Relaxed breathing is the opposite of what happens when a person is scared or angry.

Scared or angry emotions produce a sudden in-breath that is held in the upper chest with shoulders raised, accompanied by a sensation of internal pressure and contraction in the area of the middle-body diaphragm muscle area ('a knot in the stomach'). A therapist may demonstrate or act this out for the adolescent. This breath is designed to give maximum energy for the fight-or-flight response associated with adrenalin. There are lesser levels of this more extreme description. When a person feels even a little anxious the diaphragm will be tight and unrelaxed.

Explain what to expect in order to avoid unrealistic expectation or fears of failure. It is important to explain that there is a training period and that, as with any learned skill, practice and patience are required.

Use an analogy, and elaborate on it, likening the process to the learning of the motor skill of bike riding or learning to play an instrument. In learning to ride a bike, if the adolescent fell off the first time they did not say, 'That's it! I can't do that!' and put the bike away. They accepted falling off as part of the learning and they persevered despite any mistakes. Children learn, in their own time, to balance, steer, manage uneven ground, brake and go downhill, simply because they practise, they do not criticise themselves and they do not give up! All this can be said of learning to relax or meditate. As in bike riding, focus on the details of the task and the pleasure of it.

Unlike bike riding, however, being able to relax is not a skill many people have. Most people perceive relaxing as having fun with friends or watching TV or listening to music. These activities may also give pleasure and release endorphins, especially if they involve laughter. They are, however, dependent on being in a particular place or on external agents and are not necessarily available when they are needed. 'Fun' can be coloured or even turned off by a bad mood or event. Conscious relaxation and mindfulness practice is ultimately quicker in its effect and can be done anywhere independent of time, mood, place or other people.

Alert the adolescent to the possibility of an increased awareness of sensations (including pain), and that they may have thoughts and feelings they have not been aware of before. These may be pleasant or unpleasant. If they are unpleasant, it is likely they will want to avoid the experience. Learning to accept and manage these experiences is part of the learning process that occurs with support from the therapist. Removal or avoidance of unpleasant experiences is not the aim. Remind them that unpleasant experiences exist for us all on a daily basis and that it is impossible to remove them or to totally avoid them.

Provide a focus. This may be the breath, an image, proprioceptive sensations in the muscles, a biofeedback signal or the therapist's voice.

Give an understanding that rating one's performance is not helpful and that if this occurs, they should simply refocus on the stimulus suggested. (*See* Handout 8: Learning to focus in the Appendix.)

Use language carefully. For relaxation, imply feelings of muscle relaxation, such as heaviness, stillness, ease, warmth, softness. Suggest noticing or observing rather than controlling the sensations. The therapist may measure or observe this relaxation by the adolescent's posture and by their self-reported feelings.

Provide a quiet environment, at least in the initial training period, with practice later in more challenging situations where there is noise, pain or movement (sometimes called functional relaxation).

Provide an explanation that a wandering mind is normal and that re-focussing may be helpful if other stimuli such as noise, pain, or an itch occur. Point out that if conditions are not optimal it is unreasonable to expect the same result – simply observe the different conditions. Even under difficult conditions where there is no apparent effect, taking action is what counts. It is still effective to practise as it builds a belief in self-efficacy.

Structure the session with a 'way in' and a 'way out'. A 'way in' may be to habitually go through a number of steps, for example:
⊃ 'Listen or attend to your body and make it as comfortable as possible for this moment!'
⊃ 'Start to notice the feeling of air in the nostrils. Notice which parts of body move in the breathing/feel the cool air enter the nostrils/feel it gently move the tiny hairs at the entrance.'

A 'way out' of the journey may be:
⊃ 'Before ending, feel your whole body at ease/notice your breath without trying to change it. Is it different from when you began?
⊃ Begin to hear the sounds outside/notice the chair/mat you are touching/ picture the room you are in, etc.

After some practice outside the sessions, ask the adolescent to tell you how they choose to begin and end their practices. This ability to observe the body sensations and accept them is part of the process of not reacting or engaging unduly with negative sensations or thoughts.

It can be useful to describe the process as a 'journey', particularly at the end of a practice, so that there is awareness or 'mindfulness' of the process and the changed state. Ask the adolescent to observe what has changed from the beginning to the end in terms of breathing and muscles.

Establish awareness of relaxed breathing. As the diaphragm area sinks and relaxes or 'lets go', this sensation can spread to other parts of the body with each out-breath.

Relaxed breath is associated with a soft, engaged diaphragm muscle in the middle of the body. This is observable by the therapist if the adolescent is lying prone on the floor (or is lying with bent knees balanced or supported by a cushion to soften the abdominal area). It may assist awareness if the therapist or patient's hand is placed on the abdominal area with the little finger level with the navel.

Observe the adolescent for changes as they occur and use this information to structure more learning or a change of direction – reflect back observed progress. Notice:

⊃ ease with which the eyes are kept closed
⊃ the manner of ending the session
⊃ breathing patterns and changes in speed or depth; a longer out-breath denotes ease
⊃ posture and muscle relaxation, including facial muscles, jaw and lips.

It is usually easy to see if an adolescent has not practised at home because progress is usually apparent, i.e. longer out-breaths, increased focus etc.

Work out a practise schedule. A degree of intensity is required until the adolescent has 'owned' the process and is applying it spontaneously – perhaps that includes a minimum of three practices a day for at least three weeks. This may be part of a sleep strategy or a return-to-school strategy and so may need to be done before school, at school and before bed. Although the greatest experience of relaxation occurs prone, it is essential that the adolescent use the same techniques in different positions, such as seated and walking. *This ensures that it is usable in all circumstances when needed.*

Provide ongoing support and frequency of practice in the first few weeks. Weekly contact may be enough if the adolescent is practising at home. In this way, problems such as unrealistic expectations or how, where and when to make time to practise, are addressed. Once the adolescent begins to spontaneously use it when they feel it is required, verbal coaching – even by phone – may be sufficient.

o⊶ 'Yellow flags'

Managing the barriers
Difficulty closing their eyes or increased discomfort in the initial stage
It is useful to ask if they are comfortable to close their eyes. If they do not want to, suggest they focus on an object in the middle distance for as long as they need to do this; they may feel more comfortable later. If they say yes, proceed with a few breaths with eyes lowered, then try one or two with the eyes closed. If there is fidgeting or eye fluttering, stop the process and ask them for feedback on their experience. Help them identify the source of their discomfort.

It may be simple a feeling of unfamiliarity because they have never done this before. Inward contemplation may be a new experience. It is not uncommon for an adolescent to never have had the experience of simply closing the eyes – and to immediately pop the eyes open exclaiming 'That's weird!' Gently reframe the negative sensations. 'Weird' can become 'new' or 'different'. Help them observe their feeling briefly and move their focus to another sensation that is familiar, e.g. the sensation of their feet on the ground, or the breath. You may want them to verbalise that sensation. It may be sufficient for the first time to ask them to simply observe their breathing for one or two breaths.

This may serve as the basis for home practice until the next session. It may be helpful to ask the adolescent to give feedback to the therapist on what they observe, e.g. tight shoulders, tummy, etc. Suggest leaving these sensations just as they are and moving to a new observation.

Difficulty staying focused

Explain that it is normal to be distracted, particularly if they are emotionally upset, in a noisy place or if they are very uncomfortable. It can help to use an analogy. Describe this process of directing the 'mind' as being like that of a mother guiding a toddler down a hallway or path. The toddler wanders off whenever there is something distracting or interesting, the mother gently says, 'No, we are going this way.' The successful mother persists whenever the toddler wanders and the mother who doesn't want tears or a fight, does this kindly without getting cross! A cross or critical mother meets with struggle and resistance. She does not allow the toddler to have his or her way because she understands that he or she will learn how to find a direction so that mother and child are going in the same direction in a trouble-free manner.

Breaking down the process into small steps will help with either of the above problems. Limiting the number of breaths may be helpful. Instead of counting, which becomes another distraction and causes more difficulty in trying to focus, use finger movements to limit the exercise. With the hands lying flat on the lap or on the body, move one finger sideways at each breath to mark each one. In this way the exercise can be limited or increased within groups of five. Once 20 breaths have been achieved, it is likely the adolescent will feel confident to continue without this aid. It may be necessary to gradually increase the ability to focus over a number of weeks, i.e. by asking for four practices of five focussed breaths daily for one week, with an increase if the adolescent feels it possible. This is an excellent way of gauging compliance. It is usually obvious when no practice has occurred. This is an opportunity to discuss barriers and difficulties and to negotiate commitment. Reiterate the necessity of practice.

Pain becoming more noticeable

Somatising is a common feature amongst adolescents with persistent pain. These adolescents are likely to focus on negative sensations when the eyes are shut and find them intolerable. If this is not discussed prior to them closing their eyes it can be distressing for the therapist as well as for the adolescent or parent. Training and applied daily practice in mindfulness technique is essential as preparation (*see* description in this chapter).

Following the adolescent's practice, at the end of a session ask them to notice one pleasant feeling in their body. Equally important is that they acknowledge that, although the therapist may be guiding them, it is essentially their own application of focus that has makes the change, i.e. they have been willing to take some action (thus reinforcing self-efficacy).

Discomfort or difficulty breathing

If the adolescent finds that, in noticing their breath, the natural ease of breathing is disturbed or uncoordinated, it is best to leave that focus and do the 'notice five things' exercise (*see* below). It may be possible to gradually train them to briefly observe their breath at the end when they are more relaxed and to stay with that observation without attempting to change it. Muscle relaxation focus may also provide a mechanism for changed focus from breath.

A blocked nose is also a difficulty for focus on breath. Although mouth breathing is not a recommended practice because the sensation in the mouth is one of increasing dryness requiring movement of tongue or lips to moisturise it, this may be the only breath possible at times. The adolescent will identify whether mouth breathing feels increasingly difficult. If so, choose another mode of relaxation – in this instance possibly using imagery or sensations of muscle release.

Immediately reverting to an alert state following the session

An adolescent who pops open their eyes and moves suddenly following a session needs to be taught to slow down and to take the time to observe differences. For some adolescents whose normal state is one of hyper-alertness, being relaxed is unfamiliar and strange. They feel more comfortable in an alert state in early sessions. The therapist needs to assist them to take more time for reflection and observation at the end of each session. Ask them to open eyes their eyes slowly without other body movement at the end of the session. In this state of stillness, ask them to observe any differences.

No diaphragm breath observable

Assist awareness by placing therapist's or patient's hand on the abdominal area with the little finger level with the navel. Ask the adolescent to breathe deep down, filling up under the hand so that it lifts up on the in-breath. This can give a sensation of breathing deeply into the hips. Doing some regular practice of five or so deep breaths like this at the start of each session can expand a tight diaphragm muscle.

Lack of belief in the process

This can be a form of resistance to change or it can be a manifestation of a 'black-and-white' thinker who requires 'proof'. Biofeedback can provide this 'proof' in the form of visual or auditory feedback. Once the adolescent recognises the cognitive processes that produce the visible change on the screen, they are more able to recognise the body sensations that accompany it. Resistance needs to be addressed as a separate issue (*see* Chapter 4) and relaxation stopped. If a degree of acceptance is reached, mindfulness training may assist in observing resistant thoughts.

Increased awareness of unpleasant sensations, thoughts or feelings

This needs understanding and support as the adolescent is most likely to want to avoid this experience and therefore stop the practice. Having alerted them initially to the possibility of the experience of unpleasant or unwanted thoughts, sensations or feelings, it is important to invite the adolescent to speak up as these occur during a session. Some of the more common negative experiences described are likely to be nausea or dizziness, an increase in pain, or thoughts that provoke anxious feelings with an increased heart rate. It is important not to use techniques that may encourage avoidance, such as visualisations of pleasant places. It is also important to understand that the process is not aimed at changing whatever is unpleasant – though they may observe change during the process. Use mindfulness training.

The therapist can assist the adolescent to 'observe' the sensations by creating an image that *represents* the unpleasant experience. One way of doing this is to ask what it would look like in a painting – how would they paint or draw it; what colour would it have; does it move, e.g. throb or pulsate; does it have texture, e.g. prickly or bumpy; what shape is it? For example, nausea may be green, pulsating or wavy, etc. Other unpleasant internal events may be words that are terrifying, humiliating or overwhelming. These too can be observed as an image.

Here are samples of images that have arisen in sessions.

1   An adolescent with headaches described a series of rolling black cylinders that continued to roll on and on in a never-ending stream. The adolescent was able, with the breathing techniques described below, to breath into the space around the barrels, thereby diminishing their number and frequency.

2   One boy in treatment experienced a number of extremely unpleasant body sensations that occurred when he experienced the internal self-talk of 'I am an idiot'. He was able to contain and therefore 'observe' these words in a digital image on a television screen. Initially he was unable to even say out loud 'I am an idiot.' With practice he learned to say the words aloud over and over until they lost some of their power for him.

3   Pain is frequently represented in red/orange colours in various abstract shapes.

> *It is important not to supply the image for the adolescent as they must face the 'unwanted event' sufficiently to be able to identify and shape it in some way.*

> *Exposure to the experience is the first most important stage of the process of acceptance. It may need to be done in gradual stages of exposure, with discussion afterwards on their gradually increasing ability to accept the negative event – whatever it is.*

⊶ 'Yellow flags'

An adolescent who chooses not to close their eyes even after a rapport has been established and preliminary sessions have occurred can have significant issues of trust. These issues need further assessment from a psychologist or psychiatrist, especially where there is a possibility of physical or sexual abuse in the history.

An adolescent whose attention to their body is unswervingly negative, and/or who has a history of presentations of repeated illness or disability without underlying pathology, and/or a range of physical symptomatology where there is no clear diagnosis or underlying pathology may require further assessment from a psychologist or psychiatrist.

Although there is a spectrum of somatising, these are indicators of long-standing psychopathology.

An adolescent who presents with a consistently flat affect and sadness, accompanied by a focus on negative appraisals of themself and their environment, fatigue and poor sleep, may be clinically depressed and may require a referral to a psychologist or psychiatrist for assessment. If depression is suspected it is not advisable to attempt relaxation. Inward contemplation is not a positive experience for them and is likely to increase their negative mood. This person is better served by encouragement of increasing physical and social activity at least initially, until the depression has lifted.

Applying the practices

All practices are tools to allow greater function in life, they are not an end in themselves. Although they are taught usually in artificial situations such as in sessions with a therapist, it is imperative that they be applied in everyday challenging situations, e.g. going to sleep, climbing stairs, sitting or walking for a prolonged period, in the middle of a shopping centre, etc. The techniques need to be useable in many situations and should not require special equipment or environments (i.e. should not require special background music, aromas or even complete silence). The aim is to help the adolescent acquire a degree of psychological flexibility that will allow them to continue in their life and to be aware of and accept unpleasant private events. If, as suggested earlier, there is a tendency for some adolescents with pain to have low tolerance to negative thoughts and sensations and for avoidant behaviours to accompany these, it is very important that the teaching of relaxation, or the use of imagery does not encourage avoidant practices.

A therapist needs to consider for what therapeutic purpose a technique is required. It may be need for any of the following.

⊃ *Quietening the autonomic nervous system response* that is characteristic of anxiety, e.g. as in a graduated sensitisation programme where an increase in heart rate or other negative sensations – including pain – occur in situations that trigger anxiety symptoms. Use breath focus and mindfulness.

↺ *An awareness of the coexistence and transience of sensations in the body as well as acceptance of negative sensations* as in anxious, somatising or avoidant adolescents who are reluctant to accept the presence of pain. Use breath focus and mindfulness training, e.g. observe, breathe, expand and allow.

↺ *To teach psychological flexibility*, i.e. the ability to adapt and transfer focus at will from one place to another without becoming attached or fused with one. This is part of mindfulness exercises, e.g. in 'notice five things', expand on how the observing mind can travel freely and at will and that thoughts are transitory, they come and go.

↺ *For initiating sleep and muscle relaxation.* Breathing techniques with imagery and focus on muscle relaxation are useful. Pleasant imagery can assist in initiating sleep by engaging the mind. However, mindfulness needs to be practised as well, so that imagery is not an avoidant activity but simply a means of initiating sleep.

> *•Life triggers the challenges and avoidance behaviours.*
> *Practise the techniques in the life situations.*
> *This is the key to success.•*

Scripts for therapists

1 Diaphragm breathing exercise

a Lying on the floor

Remove your shoes. Loosen any tight-fitting items of clothing from around your neck or waist. Lie on your back on a firm surface (not *in* bed). You may find it more comfortable to complete the exercise in a warm room or with a blanket as your body temperature lowers when you are lying still. You may like to support your head with a pillow. It is best to lie symmetrically, with your legs out and feet slightly apart. Alternatively, you may prefer to have your knees bent with feet about hip-width apart. A pillow can be used to prop up the legs.

Close your eyes and bring your attention to your breathing. Notice the sensation of breathing in and out. Feel the air passing through the nostrils. Notice it is cool on the in-breath and warm on the out-breath. Be interested in every detail and sensation.

If you find your mind wanders, notice that it has and gently bring it back to the task. No matter how many times you need to do this, do it without judging yourself.

Place both your hands gently on your abdomen. Inhale slowly and deeply through your nose into your abdomen to push up your hands as much as feels comfortable. Your chest should only move a little. If this exercise becomes uncomfortable or makes you feel tense, just focus on your normal breathing pattern. You might like to place one hand on your chest and one hand on your abdomen and just feel your hands rise and fall (with the little finger on top of your navel).

Continue to take in long, deep, slow breaths. Focus on the feeling of breathing out; notice the feeling of softening in the abdomen as you breath out; let the sinking, softening feeling there last for as long as is comfortable. You may notice a special moment when there is no air, and that you are quite still. At this special moment even your breathing muscles are relaxed. You are at your most relaxed. Stay with that moment, watch it, allow it to stay for as long as is comfortable, i.e. until you naturally breathe in. Do not hold the air out as this will become uncomfortable. Your relaxing out-breath will gradually lengthen in this process.

Notice the changed sensation within your body when you are relaxed. Continue for as long as you like. At the end of the exercise, spend a little time appreciating the sensation of relaxation so that you can take it with you!

b In a chair or walking

You can do modified versions of the above script for sitting in a chair, or even for walking. In these positions, the experience is different so it is important not to expect the same outcome. Because the seated position squashes the abdominal area, it is more difficult to feel the diaphragm moving the lower abdomen. It is easier to feel the shoulders and ribs sinking as you breathe out, so this sensation is also a useful area for focus. If concentration is difficult, you may like to restrict your practice to just ten breaths by moving one finger for each breath. In this way you are still able to focus on the sensations of relaxing rather than trying to remember to count.

See also Handout 9 in the Appendix.

2 Mindfulness

It is important to practise mindfulness in everyday activities as well as at times when unpleasant internal events occur.

Noticing five things

This is a simple exercise to centre yourself, and connect with your environment. Practise it throughout the day, especially at any time you find yourself getting caught up in your thoughts and feelings.
- Pause for a moment.
- Notice five things you can see.
- Notice five things you can hear.
- Notice five things you can feel in contact with your body (e.g. your feet in your shoes, the air on your face, your back against the chair and the fabric of your clothes touching your legs).

This is a good exercise to use when walking to school or even in class.

Mindfulness of a task

Pick an activity you do every day. It may be cleaning your teeth, making your bed, washing the dishes. Notice every detail involved in this task. If you are cleaning your teeth, notice exactly what your toothbrush looks like as you place the toothpaste on it; its colour, the shape of the bristles, the spaces between them, then the shape and colour of the paste and the smell that comes with it. When you put it in your mouth notice the sensations that occur, the taste, temperature, saliva, your tongue, etc. If you get bored or frustrated, simply notice what you're feeling and bring your attention back to the task and the details you can notice.

Again and again, your mind will wander. As soon as you notice this, gently notice what distracted you and bring your attention back to your current activity.

This is useful to do in class if pain interrupts your concentration.

Observe, breathe, expand, allow

This exercise employs some of the breath awareness and detachment or defusion exercises described earlier. It is important to establish at the beginning that these exercises are not intended to control, remove or diminish the negative private events although they may change over time. The exercise can be used in graduated exposure programmes that increase tolerance and acceptance of them while goals or values-based actions continue.

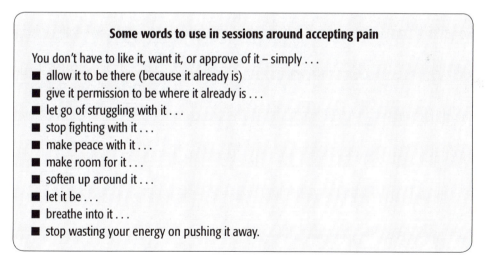

Some words to use in sessions around accepting pain

You don't have to like it, want it, or approve of it – simply . . .

- allow it to be there (because it already is)
- give it permission to be where it already is . . .
- let go of struggling with it . . .
- stop fighting with it . . .
- make peace with it . . .
- make room for it . . .
- soften up around it . . .
- let it be . . .
- breathe into it . . .
- stop wasting your energy on pushing it away.

While an adolescent is pursuing goal-based activity, they may experience any unpleasant private event (e.g. an increase in pain, or anxiety). If this would normally cause them to withdraw from the activity, suggest they do the following.

⊃ ***Observe*** the details of the sensation or thought. Notice where it is in the body; does it move, throb; does it have a definition, shape, colour or texture; write the words up on a screen?

⊃ **Breathe** into the area around the sensation or words and into the shape itself.

⊃ **Expand:** make space around it to make room for it.

⊃ **Accept** that it is there and allow it to be there, saying 'I don't like this feeling but I have room for it' or 'Its unpleasant but I can accept it' or 'Just notice it and move on.'

A useful acronym to remember the process is OBEA. (O is for observe, B is for breathe, E is for expand, A is for accept.)

See also Handout 10 in the Appendix.

Imagery or visualisation

This practice is commonly used to assist children with the acute pain resulting from medical procedures. Because it is not aimed at awareness of body sensations, it is to some extent teaching avoidance of the internal experience of pain. However, there are times in clinical practice when an adolescent may benefit from this skill, in particular when initiating sleep or when facing a medical intervention. It is worth noting that some more concrete-thinking adolescents find the use of imagery difficult.

Steps to visualisation

Choose an event or activity that is enjoyable and engaging to the adolescent. This might be making and eating a pizza, being at the beach or in a garden, walking in the country. Do not use language that implies a pretending game. When you begin, simply state the place or event or sensation as a fact, e.g. 'You are at the beach', 'Feel the warmth of the sand on your toes', etc. State that it is all right for them to answer you as you go on the journey.

Ask them to close their eyes. As this is a shared visualisation between the therapist and the adolescent, the therapist also can visualise and feel as if they are there. The therapist can ask questions about positions of items or objects if the place is known to the adolescent. They will correct you if you suggest something that does not fit with their image, or they can suggest the details of the scene, e.g. there are rocks on the beach. Use colour, texture, and temperature and body sensations to do this, 'Feel the sun on the skin.'

Find an easy flow in describing the imagery. Do not be concerned about making a mistake. Allow the description to flow easily using the present tense. If the adolescent is engaged they will fill in any gaps or modify their own image to suit.

Notice if there is emotion visible or whether muscles relax. This will depend on the subject of the imagery. If using this for sleep it is appropriate to choose one that will induce muscle relaxation rather than excitement and muscle tension. If the experience is pleasurable, it is likely that breathing will slow and muscles will relax.

Make sure there is an ending that brings the adolescent to an awareness of the here and now. Ask them to remember the room and perhaps to count backwards from five as a cue to open the eyes.

Record of practice

Instructions

This record is primarily for your benefit so you can keep track of when you have practised. Record when you have done practice at the end of each day. It can be helpful to note the time. Initially, learning relaxation/mindfulness requires a short burst of intense learning, so aim for at least three practices of any length. Regularity and frequency of practice are more important than the length of each one. If you start with one and your record shows you are gradually managing to add one more, you are on the right track. The more you do it, the better you will be at it. Build it into your daily routine and activities, for example in class, as a passenger in the bus or car or on the way to school. In particular, practise it when you notice a familiar trigger for an unpleasant sensation, thought or feeling – including when, because of pain, you want to avoid an activity that you are fit enough to do.

Record of practice

Start date: _____   *Name:* _____

DAY	UP TO 20 MINS	UP TO 5 MINS	UP TO 5 MINS	UP TO 5 MINS	UP TO 5 MINS	CHALLENGES/TRIGGERS
1						
2						
3						
4						
5						
6						
7						
8						
9						
10						
11						
12						
13						
14						

➲ Fill in days of the week.
➲ Place a tick (or the time of day) for each relaxation/mindfulness session.
➲ Record events that triggered unpleasant sensations (e.g. pain), thoughts or feelings where you used the technique in the challenges column.
➲ Full regular practice is best.
➲ Remember, relaxation takes practice, the more regularly you do it, the easier it becomes.

See also Handout 11 in the Appendix.

Further reading

Davis M, Eshelman E, McKay M. *The Relaxation and Stress Reduction Workbook*, 5th ed. New York: New Habinger; 2006.
Hayes S, Strosahl K, editors. *A Practical Guide to Acceptance and Commitment Therapy.* New York: Springer; 2004.
Kabat-Zinn J. *Full Catastrophe Living: how to cope with stress, pain and illness using mindfulness meditation.* London: Piatkis; 1990. http://www.noetic.org/research/medbiblio/ch_intro2.htm
Poppen R. *Behavioural Relaxation and Training and Assessment*, 2nd ed. Thousand Oaks: Sage; 1998.
Sadler J. *Natural Pain Relief: a practical handbook for self-help.* Dorset: Element Books; 1997.

References

1 Eccleston C, Yorke L, Morley S, *et al.* Psychological therapies for the management of chronic and recurrent pain in children and adolescents. Cochrane Review. In: *The Cochrane Library*, Issue 1. Chichester: John Wiley & Sons; 2004.
2 Kabat-Zinn J, Lipworth L, Burney R. The clinical use of mindfulness meditation for the self-regulation of chronic pain. *J Behav Med.* 1984; 8(2): 163–90.
3 Poppen R. *Behavioural Relaxation Training and Assessment*, 2nd ed. Thousand Oaks: Sage; 1998.

CHAPTER 8

Thought, words and actions

LANGUAGE AND ITS ROLE IN BEHAVIOUR

CHAPTER SUMMARY

This chapter gives an outline of the function of the internal processes of thoughts, language and images and their impact on behaviour. The importance of a case formulation and the identification of depression are stressed. Treatment is described, looking at the parental role in learning processes that include modelling, reinforcement and focus on emotion. An education process for parents is outlined and the uses of a diary to identify emotions and actions are discussed. Language that is helpful for therapists to notice in sessions is discussed and some suggestions for the use of metaphors in therapy are outlined. Examples of completed diaries are given, followed by a case study.

Background

Thoughts can take the form of words or images, kept silent and unacknowledged. These thoughts can include subjective appraisals of events and people. The same event experienced by two different people may trigger quite different appraisals. A person's interpretation impacts on their thoughts and feelings. One person who knows nothing about sharks and who is unable to swim, may picture a shark beneath the water under their boat and experience fear (a pumping heart and shakiness). This image (or thought) may produce an action of deciding not to go out in a boat again. Another person who studies sharks and pictures one under the boat may feel excited and hopeful that they may see a rare species.

Spoken words also affect our actions and the actions of others. The intention in this chapter is to assist in identifying whether thoughts (here including images) and words (spoken) help or hinder the adolescent with persistent pain. Awareness of thoughts and words is often the primary task. This chapter will look at practices to achieve this awareness.

Once again, since the bulk of research has been done in adults with chronic pain, the relevance of these findings for the adolescent population is a matter of conjecture. It has been found that an adolescent with chronic or persistent pain who is seeking help is likely to have difficulties in other aspects of their lives. They are likely to have higher levels of negative affect, fear of failure, greater use of emotion-focused avoidance coping strategies and less strong perceptions that they are socially accepted.[1]

Case formulation

A careful history and case formulation (*see* Chapter 1) will alert the therapist to areas that require attention concurrently with pain, e.g. bullying plus academic performance difficulties, plus avoidant behaviour and parental reinforcement behaviours. Allowing a place in which the adolescent can speak freely and explore these issues may also help them accept that external problems can be addressed separately and are different from the sensory experience of pain and the thoughts that accompany that sensation. Learning to recognise problems and associated negative feelings is the beginning of a positive coping strategy that seeks help from outside sources.

Clinical depression

Adolescents with chronic pain and their parents report high levels of depression.[2] It is therefore important to diagnose clinical depression if it is present. Untreated clinical depression will prevent progress in any rehabilitation programme. The signs of clinical depression are not easily separated from the symptoms that accompany persistent pain, i.e. sadness, frequent or continuous crying, an inability to see hope for the future, negative ideation, poor sleep and fatigue. These can be secondary to the persistence of the pain over time.

Pain prevents good sleep which in turn leads to fatigue, a loss of previously rewarding activities and a feeling of there being no way out of the problem. A clinician who is not a psychologist may notice any of these signs and need confirmation from a psychologist or psychiatrist in order to make a proper diagnosis of clinical depression in either the parent or the adolescent.

ᴏ⚓ 'Yellow flag'

An adolescent who is unable to articulate or who becomes unduly distressed in contemplating their values or goals may be suffering from clinical depression. In depression, feelings of hopelessness may prevent any envisaging of a positive future. An adolescent in a rehabilitation programme that becomes stalled for no obvious cause except that the adolescent is unable to carry out any of the activities asked of them may be clinically depressed.

Treatment

In a clinical setting, each adolescent is an individual with unique personal and cultural characteristics. Despite this uniqueness, it is nevertheless possible to see in the adolescent the general concepts discussed in Chapter 6: anxiety, sensitivity, fear of movement, catastrophising thoughts, and thoughts of disability, etc. The goal of treatment is to assist the adolescent to adopt patterns of behaviour that will lead them towards their valued goals (*see* Chapter 5) and to ever-increasing patterns of this behaviour that will maintain this path. It is likely that, in varying degrees and combinations, the adolescent feels ineffective in the face of their pain (self-efficacy). They are frequently withdrawn from activities as well as emotional and social experiences (avoidant coping). They show negative interpretations (beliefs), colourful language or imagery and excessive attention to pain (catastrophising and somatising). Furthermore they behave as if the pain is going to damage them when they move (fear avoidant). In short, they are likely not to be leading the life that is consistent with their values.

Thoughts, images or emotions (private events) or self-talk or automatic thinking, loosely called inner processes, can be helpful or unhelpful. Cognitive behaviour therapy (CBT) (control-focused) and contextual cognitive behavioural therapy (CCBT) (acceptance-focused) both accept the necessity for awareness of inner processes and the ability to observe them as they occur, since unhelpful inner processes may result in avoidant behaviour or maladaptive behaviours. An early study comparing acceptance-focused and control-focused treatment for an adult chronic pain population showed no difference at follow-up between the two groups, with both showing significant improvement in physical and psychosocial disability, mood and daily activity.[3]

Education

Psychological awareness varies a great deal between individuals and families. What is easily understood by some may be difficult for others. Simple explanations may help the adolescent begin a process of increasing their awareness of their thoughts and feelings. For some adolescents and parents, psychology is associated with mental illness or abnormality and there is a fear of being 'analysed'. An explanation of normal psychology can be very helpful in dispelling these fears and myths. The therapist may need to judge how much explanation and education is required to help the adolescent move forward. However, normalising the process of understanding thoughts and feelings is helpful. Choosing how to include the parent in this process and which parts of the process to follow at which time is also a matter of judgement.

Topics of relevance for education are:
1   how we can change our mind
2   how we, as humans, learn
3   the parental role
4   the relationship between thoughts and emotions (feelings)
5   feelings and body sensations
6   the power of thoughts images and words
7   unhelpful words and thoughts.

How we can change our mind

The following story based on early CBT research can be helpful to demonstrate how we acquire our beliefs, how they can change, and what might influence them.

A useful story

A group of salespeople were asked to choose from a group of items something that they would never want themselves – something they believed to be useless, ugly and generally unsellable. As part of their training they were then taught a scripted sales pitch that described the positive features of their chosen 'unattractive' item. They were then asked to sell the item, using the sales pitch they had learned. The sales pitch described how attractive and useful the item was. After two weeks of this sales activity, they were then asked how they felt about their item. Their opinions had changed, they now believed that the item was attractive and useful and they would even want to own it themselves.

Reflecting on this experiment it is possible to see that we may hold an opinion or belief, and even have 'reasons' or a rationale to support this belief. However, if we commit words and actions in a direction that is not consistent with our stated 'reasons' or 'beliefs' and, even if we don't initially believe these new words or actions, we eventually persuade ourselves and change our minds, whatever rationale we had originally constructed.

It is worth noting that the change may only have occurred because the new behaviour was congruent with a fundamental (unstated) value, which was to make money. This was reinforced whenever they sold any of their items. The essence of this experiment remains that we come to believe what is reinforced from repeated actions in the environment and thoughts and words which we repeat over time.

This story is useful to recall later in therapy at times when the behaviour required is in conflict with the adolescent's thoughts and emotions. When the salespeople were repeating their learned script when trying to sell the item, they were acting 'as if' they believed their words. The adolescent may also need to commit themselves to acting 'as if' sometimes in therapy. They may need to act 'as if' the pain or other negative emotions do not bother them, for example, when new overt action is required (i.e. staying in the classroom instead of withdrawing or attending school). Acting 'as if' can be a useful term to trigger or remind the adolescent of this story where changing overt behaviour results in changed thoughts and emotions.

Learning

There are many ways of learning. The following is an outline of what may be significant in changing behaviour associated with pain.

When we are rewarded for an action we are likely to want to do it again because we enjoy the reward. A reward may be achieving success at a task; someone praising or smiling at us; money; time spent with someone special; coming first, etc. We may not even notice the 'reward' because it is natural to do what we enjoy. The more we are rewarded, the more the behaviour is 'reinforced', and the more we are likely to do it again. Conversely, we do not want to continue those activities which are unpleasant. Naturally pain comes under this category. We get rewarded (or punished) through our relationships. Loving relationships make us feel good about ourselves. Our self-esteem is dependent on feedback from others (rewards or lack thereof) about ourselves in our environment, i.e. our skills, friendships, etc. This is how we know what sort of person we are. 'I am the sort of person that is good at . . ., has many friends . . ., is a loner . . ., is kind . . .', etc. This is information gained from other people's reflections on our behaviour. Our self-esteem is constantly fed by interactions with the environment on a daily basis. Withdrawal from activities and friendships deprives us of this feedback. If the feedback is negative, such as when bullying occurs then, unless we are able to take action that changes that feedback, self-esteem is lowered and we withdraw – thereby maintaining the cycle. (This discussion may assist in problem solving around peer relations and school policy and seeking other assistance.)

Another way in which we learn is by observing and modelling or imitating people around us. Again, we may not notice that we are doing this because it has been happening since early childhood. This happens with all sorts of behaviours and that is how family habits or cultures are built. Perhaps you have noticed yourself how your family expresses emotions or manages pain differently from another family? A child observing a mother grimacing when in pain is more likely to do the same, or a child seeing their mother holding back tears and saying 'I'm OK' and rejecting any comfort is likely to see this as what you do when you are upset.

A third way of learning is by observing and deduction, so that if two events happen repeatedly in association, it is likely that you will try to work out how this happens. You may think about the problem and reach a conclusion that satisfies you. You may conclude that one event causes the other in some circumstances but not in others. Or you learn by experience and an example may be when you look at a map and work out which is the shortest route to take but after experiencing the drive find that it actually takes longer because the traffic is worse on the shortest route. A person can work out for themselves the desired way to solve a problem having seen the outcome from other people's behaviour. 'I've seen what happens when you do X . . . And I don't want that to happen to me!'

Explore the parental role

Explain reinforcement

Positive reinforcement is a response to the adolescent's behaviour that will increase the likelihood of the behaviour occurring again. Attention for pain behaviour is a very powerful reinforcer for children. Negative reinforcement is also likely to change behaviour. This occurs when a child is bullied and they choose to avoid the bully or the place where it occurs.

Modelling

Parental influence may be considerable as models of helpful or unhelpful language and behaviours. Parents who themselves experience chronic pain may relate their child's experience to their own and personalise or share their experience with their child. Both parties are best served if the parent seeks independent ongoing treatment.

Emotions

Parents' emotions influence their children's somatic complaints and expression of pain. An adolescent may habitually and unconsciously respond to their parent's anxious words or actions around their pain. A child who has learned to become the emotional support for a parent with pathology (anxiety, depression, agoraphobia) may feel the need to help or save their parent by keeping them company at home.

For parents who have accepted the suggestions that arise from the pain physiology education session, simply informing them and coaching them through the process of what might be helpful language and behaviours is sufficient. Assisting the parent to modify their behaviour and language as models for their child and to act as a coach may be sufficient.

'Do's and don'ts' handout for the family (*see* Handout 3 in the Appendix)

It is important to gauge the appropriate time to present this handout. The timing may be appropriate after the initial pain physiology education or following any part of the following psychological education process. For some parents this advice can be very confronting. Talk through with parents whatever aspects may cause discomfort. They may believe that their child will feel they don't care about them and have abandoned them. Parents may be concerned that they are unsupportive of their child or that they won't know if their child is unwell. For some parents it is simply that they are unable to bear the feelings they experience themselves in this changed behaviour. These parents may require ongoing psychological support to understand their role in regulating their child's emotions.

It is also advisable to discuss with the adolescent how they will feel if their parent stops asking about pain as suggested. It is not uncommon for the adolescent to express relief at parents withdrawing and that this desire for independence can come as a surprise to a parent. A joint session with family members and the adolescent discussing the projected changes ensures acceptance by all parties. It is important to tailor the 'do's and don'ts' to each adolescent and parent in order to make it appropriate for their situation.

Feelings and body sensations

Normalise feelings and associated body sensations and in the process assess the adolescent's awareness of their own thoughts and feelings. Explain to the adolescent that our emotional states are generally felt in our body, i.e. we notice how we feel because we notice sensations in our body.

Ask the adolescent to describe how their body feels when they are angry. If they are unable to name their sensations, ask them what a person would do to act out being angry. If necessary act out for them, the 'look' of someone who is angry. What would an actor do – clench fists, knit the brows, lift the shoulders, take large upper chest breaths and hold them until bursting point! Elaborate on their experiences of body sensations, tight chest or middle, nausea, trembling or tense muscles, dry mouth, feeling hot or cold, etc. These body sensations are produced by the activation of the autonomic nervous system discussed in Chapter 1. Describe expressions commonly used to describe feelings, 'I felt sick with worry, I couldn't eat', 'I got butterflies in my stomach just thinking about giving my talk to the class', 'He's a pain in the neck.' Discuss other 'negative' emotions and sensations such as frustration or worry that might be part of daily life. Identify with the adolescent the times when they are likely to experience these feelings and whether they are able to tolerate them and still continue their activities or whether they avoid them. Introduce the possibility of a diary to chart their experiences. Usually they will identify one or two of these feelings they experience. Use their examples when you work with them on the thought diary chart described later in this chapter.

Revisit the pain physiology education session in Chapter 1, where thoughts that produce emotions of fear were discussed. Thoughts about danger or threat activate our autonomic nervous system and sensations occur in the body which we know as fear. If we appraise the threat as real, we are likely to act on that fear to avoid the object causing the fear. If our heart rate slows and our breathing returns to normal, we believe we have successfully avoided the threat, we have appraised the threat as nothing to worry about and have not acted in accordance with the original body sensations of threat. However, if our heart rate is maintained and our breathing and muscles remain tense, we can remain alert and watchful for continuing or new signs of threat. We become extra vigilant and anxious about any small sign.

Pain and body sensations

This cycle of hypervigilance occurs with pain. If we believe our pain is a sign of damage or disability (a threat), our autonomic nervous system will be activated. Adrenalin is released, thereby increasing pain and other negative sensations such as a thumping heart, dizziness, tight muscles, etc. Any new body sensation is interpreted as part of the threat of damage or harm. Having been alerted, we watch for more (pain, etc.) and so the cycle continues. In this scenario, *normal* body sensations are interpreted as evidence of threat causing more hypervigilance and yet more negative interpretations. Ask the adolescent to identify if there was an event that they felt so anxious about that they felt pain or other uncomfortable body sensations such as dizziness. (This information is the basis for the mindfulness meditation practice suggested in Chapter 7.)

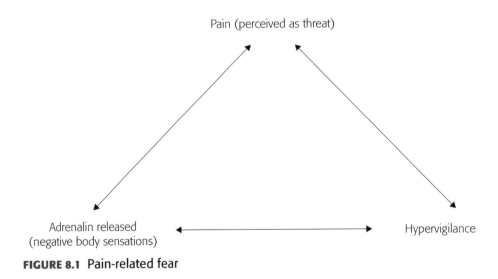

FIGURE 8.1 Pain-related fear

Acting 'As if'

Ask the adolescent if there was ever a time when they had to act against their feelings and that the action turned out to be the right decision?

Use an example as a basis for discussion, for example: 'Have you ever had to do something that is a bit scary or worrying, such as going abseiling or rock climbing, on camp? The thought of it makes you feel sick and your heart race. You want to get out of doing it but all your friends are doing it. Your friends have probably experienced the same racing heart and fearful thoughts but they have chosen to ignore these sensations. (Maybe they talked themselves through the appraisal of threat, deciding that it was safe enough.) Deciding to continue with the climb would mean acting "as if" the body sensations are not there. At the end of the climb, you would be able to say, "The climb isn't so bad after all – I wouldn't mind doing it again." The appraisal of threat is diminished by taking action, despite the body sensations and scary thoughts, i.e. by the acting "as if". However, if you choose not to continue with the climb, whenever rock climbing is mentioned it is likely that those same autonomic responses of fear will appear and you will remain afraid of doing it.'

○— 'Yellow flags'

Some adolescents are unaware of what emotional states the body sensations connect to. There may be a number of reasons why an adolescent fails to identify emotions or body sensations:
- they cannot tolerate unpleasantness or discomfort and so habitually repress or avoid them
- feelings and sensations are mysterious and therefore powerful and the adolescent may fear loss of control (*see* 'Case study: Bernie' in Chapter 10)
- the adolescent may not have the language at their disposal
- it may be that the family is one in which feelings are not expressed or recognised and words that express feelings are not used (*see* Chapter 3).

Referral to a psychologist may be required, as it is important that the adolescent learns to recognise these negative sensations and emotions as they can be the source of unhelpful avoidant behaviour.

The power of thoughts, words and images

A single word can immediately conjure up an image and a body response. Ask the adolescent if they are hungry and what their favourite food is. Did the question cause them to salivate? Imagine biting into a lemon, jumping into a freezing pool, etc.

Words and thoughts are very powerful they are based on our learning from previous experiences and conclusions we have drawn from them. If something has happened several times then we tend to expect that this will happen again. We look out for it happening again. When it does, it becomes predicable and in an unspoken way we think of it as true. We are likely to base our future decisions on the generalisation of this 'truth'. It is our 'reality'! An example to suggest to the adolescent is the different power and meaning contained in the word 'pain'. Because of their pain experiences, 'pain' is much more complicated in meaning for them (the adolescent) than it is for their friend who has experienced little pain. Our past histories have prepared us to have particular thoughts and responses that become automatic, e.g. 'I'm hopeless', 'Whenever 'X' happens I have to stop' ('X' can be pain, a feeling of failure, etc.). It is these automatic thoughts can drive our behaviour and our feelings.

We can colour the world with positive or negative interpretations and cause feelings of worry, frustration or hopelessness which, in turn, cause us to make judgements to act accordingly. This usually reinforces our interpretations, e.g. 'I'm useless, I can't even stand up without getting pain, I'd better not go out with my friends,' 'My friends don't call me anymore, I'm useless.'

The task in therapy is to learn to catch these automatic thoughts and see whether their power is positive (helpful) or negative (unhelpful). (The discussion on mindfulness meditation in Chapter 7 addresses these thoughts.)

Talk through with the adolescent the points on automatic thoughts/self-talk below.

Automatic thoughts or self-talk has several characteristics

1 They are automatic thoughts – thoughts just 'pop up' without any effort on your part. They just seem to happen. It can help to think of them as part of the running commentary on life that goes on almost constantly inside our heads while we are awake.

2 They are often distorted. They are our own *interpretations* of what is going on around us rather than facts. They are our own filtering system that reflects a variety of factors, including our beliefs in ourselves, our environment and other people.

3 They are often unhelpful – they keep you depressed, worried or frustrated and make it difficult to change.

4 They are plausible – it does not occur to you to question them. You tend to accept them as easily as an ordinary thought such as 'I feel cold – I will put a sweater on.' You may have what seem like good 'reasons' for the thought. Our behaviour is based on our automatic thoughts. We believe them, usually without question. It is very unlikely to occur to you to stand back from them and evaluate or question them.

5 They are involuntary – they can be very difficult to switch off.

Using a diary

By using a home practice book it is possible to tailor the particular thought diary to the needs of the individual. This is best done after the education process described above has been completed. Use different headings that suit the requirements. The headings may be laid out in whatever way suits the adolescent, i.e. constructed in table form or just under headings. The adolescent may enjoy constructing their own table on the computer. Examples of some formats are to be found in the Appendix (*see* Handout 12).

Explain the reason for keeping a diary (to be aware of their thoughts and to help them decide what thoughts will be helpful in taking new, values-based actions).

Identify the triggers and use these as headings:
- physical sensations (change in pain, shakiness, tension in stomach, etc.)
- thoughts (interpretations, judgements, beliefs, criticisms, etc.)
- emotion (frustration, anger, sadness, worry, fear, etc.)
- actions (what did you actually say or do, or feel like saying or doing?)
- behaviour (what did you do?)
- consequences (what happened as a result of the behaviour?)
- alternative behaviour (what would you like to do differently next time?).

It may be necessary to break this process down to small steps to begin with.

Stage one
1 First identify an event that has recently produced unhelpful behaviour, negative emotions or sensations.
2 Ask the adolescent to recall and record thoughts that happened at that time.
3 Ask the adolescent to record only thoughts or emotions when a similar event happens again.

Stage two
1 Work with the record of thoughts and emotions produced by the adolescent.
2 Discuss actions, behaviours, consequences.

Stage three
1 Discuss alternative actions referring to previous values-based work and goals.

For some, the recognisable trigger for catching their thoughts will be an increase in pain. For others, emotional distress will trigger the first entry into the diary and the reflection on the accompanying thought. A discussion of which emotions the individual recognises most easily is important. It will also be important to reiterate the habitual nature of the feelings and thoughts, i.e.

they will recur, and they may feel like nothing much or even nonsense. Usually there are more than one, e.g. frustration, worry or sadness, hopelessness (related to depression). For some, it is important to place the emotion in the context of an event or place. For some, part of the self-management may entail nominating action other than the reframed thought, such as activating planned withdrawal from class.

Sometimes in a session it is possible to observe an adolescent experiencing discomfort. This is a valuable moment to reflect back what you observe and to ask if they are aware of their sensations in their body or their thoughts at that moment based on the headings outlined.

To start with, just associating the thought or the emotion with the pain or event is sufficient. Practising to catch the trigger at the time it occurs rather than hours later is important. The notebook therefore needs to be portable and to be kept constantly on the person at times when distress may occur. Encouragement at this stage is essential as the process may feel artificial.

The second stage is to examine the negative thought, emotion or sensation. It may be necessary to clearly distinguish between an emotion, a thought and a sensation.

Many adolescents need to do this diary work for a very short time only as they are able to start observing their thoughts and recalling the context in which they occurred quickly once the process is shown to them. Mindfulness training is helpful for this observation and for reaching a degree of detachment from the thoughts and the possibility of behaviour that is not prescribed by the thoughts, i.e. instead of withdrawing when pain increases, they are able to continue with an activity using breathing as a way of allowing this to happen.

Helpful questions for unhelpful thoughts

- Is this thought in any way useful or helpful?
- Is this an old story? Have I heard this one before?
- What would I get for buying into this story?
- Could this be helpful, or is my mind just babbling on?
- Does this thought help me take effective action?
- Am I going to trust my mind or my experience?

⚬━ 'Yellow flags'

An adolescent who reports in the diary only feelings of hopelessness and who shows flat affect, cries frequently and who has withdrawn from most social interactions is likely to require professional assessment for clinical depression.

An adolescent who finds it difficult to conceptualise abstract ideas may find it more useful to use simple flash-cards provided by the therapist using catch phrases they relate to.

An adolescent who finds it difficult to accept their imperfections or finds making mistakes threatening will find this process of looking at 'errors' difficult. They usually lack the ability to reflect on their imperfections and resist this process. These young people will be better served by referral for longer-term therapy to a psychologist or psychiatrist.

Some thoughts about thoughts

- Thoughts are merely sounds, words, stories, bits of language, passing through our heads.
- Thoughts may or may not be true. We don't have to automatically believe them.
- Thoughts may or may not be important. We can pay attention only if they're helpful.
- Thoughts are not orders. We don't have to obey them.
- Thoughts may or may not be wise. We don't automatically follow their advice.

Language for the clinician to notice
Some powerful words seem just a habit but may result in negative feelings. Some examples are given below.

never, always, forever, no-one, everyone
'This will *never* get better,' 'It's *always* like this.'

These words describe extreme states with no room to improve or change; they denote feelings of hopelessness and being stuck.

the worst, the most horrible, killing me, etc.
These words exaggerate emotions or sensations or situations (catastrophise), creating an emotional pendulum with no middle ground.

should, ought and must
These words imply strong expectations or blame, or infer that responsibility belongs to others. For example:

'This *shouldn't* happen, it's not fair,' 'They *ought* to be able to fix this.'

These denote disappointment anger, frustration or powerlessness and, by implication, 'There's nothing I can do, its life/the doctor's job and they have failed.'

The 'Yes/But' position
'But' is a barrier to functioning when used in the second part of a sentence. 'I really want to go to school but it is very hard just now.' The second half of the sentence indirectly contradicts the first half. The feeling is of doubt and conflict of interest. When an adolescent or parent include 'but' as part of their

solution it is likely they are actually unwilling or resistant to proceed in the 'agreed' direction. It can be helpful to reflect back the frequent use of 'but'. A helpful experience can be to substitute 'and' for 'but' and notice the different feeling that results. This can be done as a play dialogue where the therapist makes a number of statements that the adolescent must answer and include 'but' and then make the substitution. The changed feeling state is clarity of what is agreed and openness to the possibility to solving the problem. It allows the adolescent to feel what it's like to have other possibilities.

'You/I'

Using 'you' where the first person pronoun 'I' would normally be used to describe an experience that includes emotions, is a way of avoiding the full experience of the (usually negative) feelings engendered by the event. 'When you are at school and you can't do sport, you feel excluded' is a description once removed from the emotion. It does not 'own' the emotion as in 'When I am at school and I can't do sport, I feel excluded.' Ask the adolescent to reword it. Use a mindfulness exercise then reflect on what she/he observed.

'She/We'

It is often an indication of an enmeshed relationship when a mother habitually uses 'we' when speaking about their child. It is often noticeable in an initial assessment. A mother may say of her child 'We are not feeling so good today,' meaning 'My child/Mary is not feeling so good today,' or 'We have a lot of trouble with our maths.' It may take some time before enough understanding and trust has been established to allow reflection on the frequency and meaning of this usage with a parent.

'I tried!'

'Mistakes' and 'bad days' are a natural part of any learning process. This can be difficult for an adolescent who has perfectionist traits to accept. The use of positive language is important in the process of pain management. Never let the adolescent use the word *'try'* as it implies effort without effectiveness, i.e. 'I *tried* (but failed!)'. It usually means they are *not committed to or believing in* the process at this point. Their behaviour may not reflect their actual feelings. They may be just doing what they are told because they have a need to please or they have a self-concept that entails being 'well behaved'. It is a good idea to talk about the adolescent's non-belief as acceptable – even to be expected at the beginning of the process. This is a fitting subject for a 'mindfulness' exercise (*see* Chapter 7). Use of positive language is likely, over time, to create a positive belief. It can be useful to describe the simple experiment described in Chapter 6 that demonstrates this transition from non-belief to belief in our words. Watching the hidden or unconscious use of persuasively negative interpretations is essential, especially in the sensitive early phase of learning a new skill. Intercept this 'try' word early and assist the adolescent to understand that the **act** of taking action is the **success** and that having pre-conceived expectations about outcome (pain relief) leads to feelings of failure. Making light of it avoids any blaming or failure. Suggest that you have a box in your room in which you collect this 'try' word and at this point there are lots and lots of 'try's' in the box because it is such a commonly used word and that there have been so many people before them also needing to discard this word! The box will be eventually given to the 'thought police' for latter shredding. The 'thought police' image was one adolescent's humorous inter-pretation of the process of reframing thoughts and words.

Stories

As mentioned before in describing self-esteem, we learn about ourselves through family stories that are repeated. Sometimes these stories are not helpful as they type-cast the adolescent. It may be a story resulting from one significant event or from a series of events that the family chooses to identify with one member. 'She's the strong one,'or 'She's always been the sick one.' These stories are not necessarily true and they can imprison a person who – despite other evidence to the contrary of the main story – continues to wear a label. The 'strong one' may benefit from allowing others to help; others may presume she doesn't need help when she does. The 'sick one' may want to be healthy.

A therapist can assist in this process working with parents, by looking at events and seeing if any other interpretation is possible or working with the adolescent assisting them to assert how they want to be seen. It is possible to rewrite these stories.

Metaphors

In therapy either the therapist or adolescent may introduce a metaphor as a way of describing a process or idea. A metaphor can succinctly summarise a feeling, a process or concept and is sometimes an easier form of communication than an elaborate description. It can be useful to pursue this metaphor by elaborating on it or referring to it in later sessions as a shorthand way of reinforcing the concept. Metaphors can be shared between treating clinicians and parents for further reinforcement and consistency for the adolescent. (For some populations, such as the autism/Asperger spectrum of diagnosis, or head-injured people or concrete thinkers, metaphors are too abstract and therefore not suitable.) The appropriateness and significance of a metaphor is probably culturally determined so it is most useful if they arise naturally in therapy between therapist and adolescent. However some examples that have arisen from clinical cases are described below.

1 Being the driver of your own vehicle

When pain is in charge, possibly at the beginning of therapy, pain is behind the driver's wheel, choosing which direction and how fast to go. The aim of therapy is to have you (the adolescent) in the driver's seat so that you choose which direction to go, you get behind the driver's wheel and operate the steering and brake. The pain may still be in the car in the passenger's seat and trying to tell you what to do, but you do the steering. In time the pain may end up in the back seat or even in the boot!

2 **Create your own library**
Mick was a 15-year-boy with general body pain, and had also been diagnosed in the past with an obsessive condition. He found it hard to let his thoughts and anger go. He had been advised in therapy not to repress his thoughts; he worried that if he let his anger go after an event that triggered anger, he would be repressing his thoughts. He came up with the idea that each event that caused him to feel angry was like a book in a library. The book belonged in the library so he didn't have to try to get rid of it; it was, after all, already written. Just as the event had happened and was stored in his memory. The book was a permanent part of the library. However, although he might open the book from time to time he could close it and replace it on the shelf. This was the way Mick accepted the return of unwanted thoughts but he understood it was OK to move on with writing a new book.

3 **Shock absorbers** (*see* 'Case study: Jake' below)

4 **Pain as a shield**
After some time in therapy, Mona, a 13-year-old girl who was school phobic recognised that she used her pain as a shield. It protected her from having to face life events which caused her anxiety at school. It was a metaphor for avoidance as it enabled her to not look at anything that was on the other side. In this way she did not have to feel the unpleasant feelings and thoughts when faced with the classroom or playground. (*See* 'Case study: Mona' in Chapter 1.)

5 **A barometer**
Alice, a 12-year-old borderline intellectually challenged girl with Asperger's syndrome, who had previously injured her foot, developed the habit of walking with her heel off the ground whenever she was stressed. Her mother, who was initially convinced that this was a recurring physical injury, learned to understand that the raised heel was a 'barometer' of her daughter's stress and that when this occurred she needed to seek assistance from the school counsellor, usually because of social problems at school.

6 **The unwanted neighbour** (*see* 'Case study: Jake' below)

Case study: Jake

Jake was a 12-year-old boy, the only child of parents who had lost a child at birth prior to Jake's birth. He was a tall boy, an 'A' student known for his responsible behaviour by teachers and for his role with friends who sought his advice for problems. He was school captain and student representative on school council in his final year of primary school. Jake initially presented with pain in his left heel. No underlying pathology was discovered. Jake's father was attentive and respectful of him, frequently accompanying him to appointments. He had recently started to take Jake to the local gym with him. He described Jake as very close to his mother. Jake's mother agreed with her husband's assessment, the closeness demonstrated by constantly focusing on and gazing at her son, and her emotional lability when discussing his pain. She frequently corrected his behaviour in many small ways. 'Open the door for the doctor . . . Say thank you . . . pick up that paper for X . . .,' etc. She described her son as 'perfect', except for this strange walk he had developed.

For some months, pain had prevented Jake from placing his foot on the ground. At this time he stopped all physical activity such as running or sport. Over some months the pain diminished but he developed the habit of walking with his left knee stiff. Nine months of physiotherapy failed to correct his walk as Jake would fall whenever he bent his knee. He had good muscle strength and freely bent his leg when sitting. He was assessed by a psychiatrist who felt there were underlying family issues that the family was unwilling to address. Jake began to complain of pain in his left hip which he believed was damaged. This was how he explained his straight leg to his peers. Again, no underlying pathology was found. Jake was referred initially to the occupational therapist as this was acceptable 'physical' treatment from the mother's perspective. The father accepted that Jake's problem was 'in his head'. Occupational therapy consisted initially of a joint family education session on the physiology of pain and the relationship between thoughts and emotions. Jake's mother was seen individually for a discussion on what behaviour of hers would be helpful for her son. She became upset in this process as she believed Jake would feel abandoned by her. At this point she agreed to see a psychologist to help her deal with the feelings she was struggling with. The psychologist continued to see her over some months. During this time, Jake's mother began to recognise her role in Jake's difficulties and how she could regulate her emotions for Jake's benefit. Jake's mother described the new understanding of this role in a metaphor, as being 'a shock absorber' for Jake.

Jake continued to see the occupational therapist who worked with him to articulate his goals. Sessions were spent in the park in the street, running and walking. These graduated exposure techniques with mindfulness practices assisted Jake to become aware of his negative emotions and thoughts and the struggle he had set up for himself in attempting to avoid them. Frequently Jake would experience pain in his heel, leg or hip at times when he was required to observe the thoughts he found unacceptable. Once he recognised this pattern, he learned to continue with the action despite the thoughts. Jake created the 'unwanted neighbour' metaphor to describe the struggle he was having with the thoughts he did not want to have. He was aware of his unwillingness to give up his struggle with his 'unwanted neighbour'. He understood his efforts to avoid the negative experiences were unsuccessful as they continued to recur despite his efforts. When they did occur, he would struggle against them, trying to make them disappear. He was asked how it would be if he didn't struggle but allowed them to come and then simply not engage with them when they came: he would allow them to be there while he would continue to act in the direction he wanted. He likened this to having a nasty neighbour who picked a fight and shouted at him every time he left the house and that this shouting was upsetting. If he shouted back at the neighbour to stop, the neighbour continued anyway. It was time wasting and eventually made him stay inside his house even when he really wanted to be able to go out to see friends. Instead of engaging with the neighbour and fighting, he could acknowledge he was there and simply walk past him even if the neighbour shouted abuse at him. In time, if he did not engage with the neighbour, but simply noted his presence, the neighbour might simply give up shouting. If he argued with this hated neighbour, the arguments got worse and he felt more afraid and trapped.

TABLE 8.1 Completed diary

INCIDENT OR ACTIVITY	BODILY REACTION	EMOTIONS OR FEELINGS	THOUGHTS	ACTION	ALTERNATIVE ACTION	ALTERNATIVE THOUGHT
Scenario 1 Put-down by another student or teacher Scenario 2 Can't understand school work and unable to ask for help	Throbbing in head (this may be noticed only later or even not associated at all) Faster, tighter breathing Face goes red Heart beats faster Muscles tense Shaky	(These may be hard to find at first) anger hurt feelings scared	'This is terrible' 'I am no good at anything' 'This is the worst pain' 'I can't cope' 'Perhaps I have a growth that no one has found	Go home in pain	Briefly withdraw from class to do relaxation Mindfulness, slow breathing Seek help from teachers/ friends/ counsellor Refocus on moment	'They are only words' 'That person has the problem' 'I can cope with the pain by taking action rather than resting' 'Going home won't solve the problem' 'I can do different things (like breathing distracting, etc.)'

TABLE 8.2 Completed thought diary

INCIDENT OR ACTIVITY	BODILY REACTION	EMOTIONS OR FEELINGS	THOUGHTS	ACTION	ALTERNATIVE ACTION	ALTERNATIVE THOUGHT; % BELIEF
Sitting in maths class At home playing with the dog	Throbbing in head Leg pain Tense stomach	frustrated, annoyed sad or worried	'Its not fair' 'Why me?' 'It's never going to go away' 'I wish it would just disappear' 'Now I won't be able to try out for the team/ go out with friends' 'This is hopeless, I am no good at anything anymore' 'This is killing me, it's like a knife stabbing me' 'I won't be able to cope' 'Perhaps I have a growth that no one has found'	Ring Mum and go home Withdraw to bedroom and cry Refuse invitation to go out with friends' Refuse friends invite in case I have pain Don't move just in case	Use relaxation in class or in withdrawal room Write in diary to reframe thoughts Seek help from teachers about homework Talk to friends about what I need, i.e. to walk slowly or sit down more Talk to counsellor Distraction: visualisation listen to music play with the dog ring up a friend Accept the invitation but for a shorter time or paced activity	'I know what to do to help myself (like breathing distracting, minding my language, etc.)'; 5% 'Nobody says life is fair, but I can learn to cope with the pain by taking action' 'Going home/ resting/withdrawing – won't solve the problem'; 50% 'I can take some control by . . .' 'When I do my exercises I am taking control'; 20% 'I am the only one who can do this'; 90% 'Asking *why* doesn't help me act'; 60% 'Wishing won't help me choose what action to take' 'This pain isn't damage'; 100%

Case study: Louise

Louise was a 14-year-old girl with one younger brother. Her father was a TV director and spent extended periods of time away from home. Her mother maintained the family home in his absence but had suffered from depression at various times during Louise's life, including after her birth. She was currently on anti-depressant medication. Louise's father was a diabetic requiring daily injections of insulin. Louise went to a private school and had been extremely active particularly in dance and competitive aerobics prior to presentation to a clinic for chronic daily headache. She had only been attending school three days a week, staying at home with her mother watching TV for the other days. She had withdrawn from a number of her normal social events with friends. Louise complained of constant headache, exacerbated by attendance at particular classes at school – these classes were her least favourite classes of Mathematics, French, English and Geography. She reported a feeling of 'pressure' during these classes that she did not experience in her favourite class, Drama. There was considerable disbelief from her teachers as Louise was seen to be happy with her friends and in Drama. She seemed inconsistent to some of her teachers who made comments which Louise perceived as nasty.

Initially, Louise and her mother were given a session on pain education which included focussing on the negative effect of attention on pain. Goals were set with Louise's mother present. Louise clearly stated that returning to school full time was not her goal, but that we could include it as it was her mother's and father's goal. Her mother was counselled in ways in which she could be helpful; she had felt she had not coped with Louise and was relieved that others were taking on the problem, especially the management of getting Louise to school. She had felt it necessary to defend Louise in the face of the school's apparent disbelief of her daughter's 'sickness' as it was called in the family. In a joint session with her mother and Louise the notion of 'being sick' was addressed. Louise's mother was happy to consider different language and behaviour around pain, Louise was more reluctant. In individual session with a counsellor, Louise's mother talked about her discomfort in carrying out the different behaviour that included not asking about the pain; she felt she was being uncaring and neglectful. An education session was arranged for the father to attend when he was available. A school programme was commenced that was based on a contract with Louise and her teachers. It included some of her less favourite subjects. She commenced a thought diary that revealed a consistent emotional state of hopelessness and the subsequent need to withdraw from class and to cry in the toilets. Louise was taught mindfulness strategies to manage the physical sensations of 'pressure' she described. She was able to withdraw from class and practise breathing techniques. Louise's affect remained flat in most sessions including the psychologist's session. In these she began to reveal her feelings of depression and her fear of expressing these to her family because of her mother's depression. She did not want her depression revealed to her parents or school. Her sessions with the occupational therapist were around goals she had set, including her problems in managing at school. In all sessions, Louise only spoke of 'pressure' – the description of headache was only mentioned when the 'threat' of an increase in school hours was presented. Her hours were non-negotiable but reflected a graduated exposure to perceived threat.

On the return of her father, Louise was visibly happier and very engaged with her father to the exclusion of her mother to whom she was rude or whom she simply ignored. A joint pain-education session with her father and mother was conducted. During this session her father reported that although he agreed with everything the clinic was doing, he had a problem in not attending to Louise's pain. He felt there was a danger of Louise feeling abandoned and that it was important that she knew that he was there for her. When he saw her 'alone in her pain', he felt it was necessary to acknowledge her sickness. Louise's mother who had by this time had several sessions of individual counselling, offered alternative actions to her husband in the session. It was agreed that he would benefit from individual counselling to understand his feelings around Louise's pain. The treating team's observation was reflected back to the parents, i.e. that that despite both parents reporting a happy family life, there appeared to be disunity in parenting style. Joint sessions for the parents were suggested.

As treatment progressed for Louise, it was apparent that there was considerable security and reinforcement of her avoidance behaviour for her in being 'sick'. At one point after the session discussing sickness, she asked her mother (at home) whether she was sicker than her father. To which her mother reportedly replied, 'No darling, your father is more sick because his illness is life threatening' and the implication was – 'your illness is not'! In this way she again inadvertently reinforced Louise's 'illness' state. Louise's mother, who apparently did not understand that she done this, reported the event simply because she 'wondered why Louise had asked this question out of the blue'. Over time, Louise returned to full-time school. She and her family required long-term therapy for what was longstanding psycho-pathology that had surfaced around reported daily headaches.

Comment

Pain in the form of a headache had served this adolescent well in avoiding feelings of fear and worry in her school situation. She had multiple and longstanding problems that were maintained by her parents' unconscious reinforcement of her thinking and behaviour. The parents also had a fear of their daughter's negative thoughts and experiences, leading to unworkable attempts on their part to control the situation.

Further reading

Asmundson GJG, Vlaeyen GWS, Crombez G, editors. *Understanding and Treating Fear of Pain.* Oxford: OUP; 2004.

Knost B, Flor H, Braun C, *et al.* Cerebral processing of words and the development of chronic pain. *Psychophysiol.* 1997; **34**(4): 474–81.

Siegel DJ. *The Developing Mind: towards a neurobiology of interpersonal experience.* New York: Guilford; 1999.

References

1 Merlijn VPBM, Munfeld JA, van der Wouden JC, *et al.* Psychosocial factors associated with chronic pain in adolescents. *Pain.* 2003; **101**(1–2): 33–43.
2 Eccleston C, Crombez G, Scotford A, *et al.* Adolescent chronic pain: patterns and predictors of emotional distress in adolescents with chronic pain and their parents. *Pain.* 2004; **108**(3): 221–9.
3 Geiser CS. *A comparison of acceptance-focused and control-focused psychological treatments in a chronic pain treatment center* [dissertation]. Reno: University of Nevada; 1992.

CHAPTER 9

Becoming fit

A FITNESS REGIME, PACING AND MANAGING BARRIERS

CHAPTER SUMMARY

This chapter teases out the various levels and needs for becoming fit, and identifies steps required to achieve this. Pacing is discussed in this context, including managing over-doers, how to present pacing, the management of a setback to an adolescent and suggestions for using graphs to record progress. Difficulties in body mechanics secondary to the pain are addressed and some physical treatments commonly used to address these are described. Suggestions for the management of pain during exercise are made as well as how to keep up fitness levels post-intervention. Barriers to continuing success are considered, with possible solutions. A case study illustrates some of the issues raised in the chapter.

Background

Where activity is restricted due to pain, the restriction is a predictor of depression. In adolescents in particular, it is restriction of activity rather that the pain itself which mediates the depression.[1] Getting back to activity is essential for an adolescent, as it is their pathway to their intellectual, social and psychological well-being.

The expression 'I am going to get fit!' is often used, inviting the questions, 'Fit for what activity?,' 'What does it mean to be 'fit'?,' 'Is there such a thing as enough – or too much?' This chapter will address some of the questions that may arise for the adolescent with persistent pain. It is designed to offer guidelines for the pain clinician, whose background may not be in physical therapy, for helping the adolescent to increase general physical function. It also addresses some of the issues that arise for physical therapists in managing an adolescent with persistent pain. It is not a substitute for the specialist treatments, exercises or other therapy for injury or disease provided by physiotherapists, occupational therapists, osteopaths and other physical therapists.

The chapter is a natural progression from the previous ones that have addressed motivation and goal setting, what to do with the pain during move-ment, and mindfulness techniques. Being motivated and having direction, as discussed in Chapter 4, does not in itself guarantee a successful outcome for goals, no matter how carefully they are articulated. Adolescents may have reached this 'action' stage before and failed to bring their goals to fruition, thus reinforcing the pattern of fear and anxiety about movement. It is therefore of great importance to successfully carry their goals forward without failure and consequent disappointment.

Understanding the hierarchy of what activities would provoke most fear or anxiety in the adolescent is essential in any analysis of why earlier attempts have not succeeded. Equally important is analysing the task and the adoles-cent's ability to pace themself. The management of persistent pain is a complex process involving, amongst other things, the adolescent's relationships, past learning, thinking processes, beliefs, and even sleep. Addressing these past contributing factors **in conjunction with** increasing general physical function and fitness levels is fundamental to the adolescent establishing their belief in their ability to act on managing their pain – i.e. their self-efficacy.[2]

Fit for what?

Fit for competitive sport? Fit for playing around in the backyard with friends, or fit for a day/week at school? For many adolescents with persistent pain lasting many months, it has been a downward spiral of decreasing physical activity. This spiral usually involves a decrease in strength, cardio-vascular function and endurance. They have become de-conditioned to the extent that they are unable to manage basic functions like climbing stairs at home or school, walking in the school yard, shopping, for some, even walking unaided around the house.

In managing a return to function in pain management, it is sufficient to begin the journey and show that a positive end is possible, providing the rules of the journey are followed. Understanding this as a process teaches enduring skills that the adolescent can continue to implement independently. Seemingly unimaginable goals (such as competitive sport) then become a possibility in the future.

An adolescent at presentation may have a goal of returning to competitive sport but be unable to walk for longer than a few minutes. Providing the cause of this dysfunction is simply physical deconditioning, a generalist therapist may be able to assist in helping the adolescent begin their journey, helping them to increase basic physical tolerances (for sitting, standing, walking, stair climbing, jogging, etc.), in the process decreasing down-time and increasing up-time. (Down-time being time spent sitting, reclining or sleeping and up-time being time spent standing, walking or using the legs in action.) It is possible to use an 'up-timer' device to record up-time. Data from this can be graphed or recorded as progress or compared with data from the normal population.[3] As mentioned in the previous chapter, breaking goals down to achievable levels is essential in this process.

The aim of becoming fit is to increase endurance or the ability to do more for longer. Increasing endurance primarily works the cardiovascular system and will result in an increase in heart rate, being out of breath and probably becoming pink in the face. Some of these symptoms can be interpreted as fear and may trigger anxious thoughts in an anxiety-prone adolescent or their parent. It is important to identify these before a programme of fitness starts and to teach mindfulness as part of the exercise programme (*see* Chapter 7).

Steps to becoming fit

- ⊃ Clarify medical status with treating practitioner.
- ⊃ Clarify adolescent and family beliefs about the causes of pain – educate about the physiology of pain and diagnosis as well as other sources of pain such as that associated with muscle tightness or hypermobility (*see* Chapter 1).
- ⊃ Educate the adolescent and parents on the signs of increasing cardiovascular output, i.e. red face, puffing and pumping heart.
- ⊃ Check that all parties are prepared for the 'action' stage (*see* Chapter 5).
- ⊃ Teach pain-acceptance skills (*see* Chapters 6 and 7).
- ⊃ Assist adolescent in finding helpful thinking (*see* Chapter 8).
- ⊃ Assist parent in helpful behaviour around their child's pain (*see* Chapter 3).
- ⊃ Set goals (*see* COPM or GAS, Chapter 5).
- ⊃ Explain pacing (*see* overleaf).

➲ Analyse the task to establish basic abilities required to make up the whole goal, e.g. daily school attendance requires: the ability to sit for 30–40 minutes, to walk for 15 minutes, to remain upright for 8 hours for 5 consecutive days.

➲ Identify baselines of performance for each activity; this can be done on gym equipment or by fast walking, sitting, etc.

➲ Increase the degree of intensity so that heart rate and breathing increase during the exercise. If a heart monitor is available, the training zone is between 60% and 80% of maximum heart rate.

➲ It is unlikely that the recommended 20–30 minutes of the training zone heart rate is possible initially so start with the measured baseline and gradually build up to the training zone. It is then possible to increase the goals incrementally and systematically.

➲ Identify a method of recording activity that suits the preference of the adolescent (graphs, computer-based record, hand notebook, digital counter, stopwatch, up-timer, etc.).

Pacing

Although pacing is recommended as a core strategy in resuming activity it remains a poorly researched technique in pain management.[4] It is a term frequently used as a strategy for managing activity in chronic pain, particularly in the adult pain population. Pacing is used as a mechanism to prevent the overdoing of activity with associated increase in pain that would otherwise result in an inability to maintain normal activity levels, i.e. an overactivity/underactivity cycle. It is designed to prevent flare-ups of pain after activity. The strategy generally refers to adapting the speed or intensity or frequency of activity by the individual to enable them to complete a task without negative consequences. Usually this means slowing down, breaking tasks or activity down to smaller pieces, taking rest breaks or doing less at one time. It is associated with 'listening' and responding to the signals from the body rather than pushing on despite feeling tired or an increase in pain.

Pacing is also used in the training of athletes or even during the running of a race. Here the term describes something similar; listening to the limits of the body and not overdoing training (or speed in a race) that would lead to an inability to maintain their level of performance and to fall behind. A good term to describe this is the 'crash-and-burn' syndrome (i.e. crashing through and burning out). In athletic training, however, pacing by necessity involves *increasing* performance. It is this additional notion of increasing performance that is also included in pacing as discussed here.

Drawing this graph (*see* Figure 9.1) on paper or board for the adolescent makes it clear that the sum of the arrows at the top, representing full activity time, is far less than the sum of the arrows at the bottom representing 'down-time' of no activity. The level of 'down-time' is also on a downward path, with

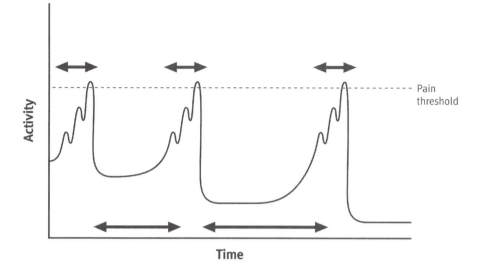

FIGURE 9.1 An overdo-er: activity without pacing

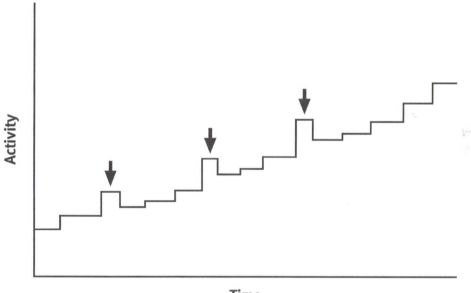

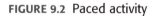

FIGURE 9.2 Paced activity

the second down-time registering less activity than the first. Furthermore, no progress of additional 'up-time' activity is apparent.

In Figure 9.2 the activity level starts at the same place and slowly progresses with times for consolidating and maintaining the level. The flat levels are the times when the level remains steady to make sure the last increase is sustainable over time. The arrows represent times when the increase is too much to sustain and the activity is dropped back to enable smaller increases again.

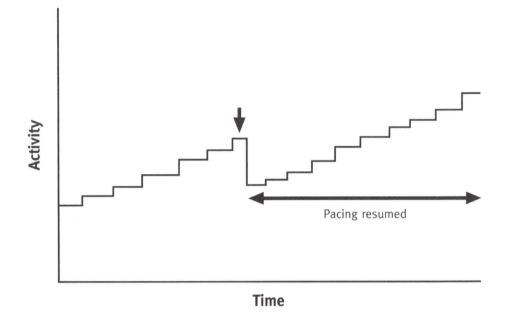

FIGURE 9.3 Managing a setback

There may be days when the level drops back, perhaps due to illness or lack of practice (*see* arrow in Figure 9.3), creating the irregularities in the graph. It is important that the same stepped progress is maintained from the point at which the dropping back occurred. It is likely that the former level will be achieved quicker than it was the first time, as the second arrows indicate when compared with the first. It is most important to point out in these graphs that at no point does the activity become excessive, nor does it drop back to full down-time. More importantly, one can make a prediction that if the steady progress is continued those high (unmaintainable) levels of 'up-time' visible in the graph of the unpaced over-doer will now be reached and be maintained.

For an adolescent able to understand graphs, starting them off on their own graph for their particular goal can be very rewarding.

These graphs need not be for a single function such as for walking. A graph may be multipurpose and include a second or third line designated with different colours. These may record, for example, a decrease in time spent on the couch or – as in the example of Bernie – a measure of increased time spent wearing articles of clothing initially found to be difficult because of allodynia, e.g. shoes, long trousers, etc.

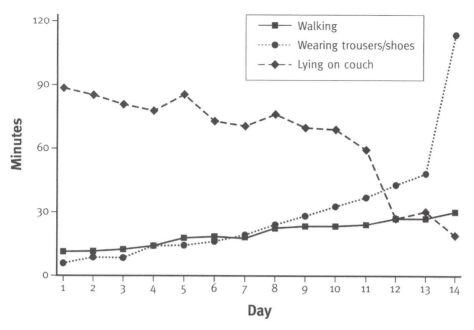

FIGURE 9.4 Combining activities: walking, lying down, wearing trousers

⊶ 'Yellow flag'

Pacing is the key to improvement in particular diagnoses, such as complex regional pain syndrome (CRPS) and other longstanding conditions like fibromyalgia and chronic fatigue.

It is a clinical observation that both CRPS and fibromyalgia can be associated with high-achieving adolescents, often in both academic and sporting arenas. The management of all these conditions requires gradual increase of regular activity. Taking the high-achieving or competitive personality into account, close monitoring of paced activity is essential to avoid flare-up of their symptoms. Understanding that there may be triggers other than over-doing activity is essential to manage relapse. (These may be a recurrence of an event associated with the original injury, such as bullying or academic challenges.) Values-based work (*see* Chapter 5) or psychological counselling may help manage inflexible behaviours or perfectionist traits. Adolescents who have strong perfectionist tendencies may require psychological help.

Body mechanics secondary to pain

It cannot be assumed that an adolescent has had adequate physical assessment nor that they or their parents understand the mechanisms at work in the adolescent's body. In the 'Steps to becoming fit' above, it is suggested that the current medical status be clarified. While this is essential in order to understand how to proceed in physical rehabilitation, clarifying whether an increase in activity is recommended or whether it is likely to exacerbate an injury is not the same as identifying the secondary consequences of pain, the impact on the whole body, post injury or pain. Muscle weakness and imbalance can occur due to longstanding disuse or movements and postures that are assumed in order to protect against pain. These lead to longstanding poor habits of body use, fatigue and pain secondary to the original pain.

Careful assessment, usually by a physiotherapist, of whole body function is required to identify areas that require attention in treatment. Treatment may be exercises targeting non-injured areas, correcting muscle imbalance or increasing strength in order to minimise upgrading pain secondary to the original area of injury or pain. It is unlikely that a graded increase in activity such as walking is likely to succeed if the adolescent's body mechanics are contributing to pain. In other words, the more they walk, the more pain they will feel due to incorrect use of the body. This pain can become confused with and even become more significant than the original source of pain.

Non-pharmacological physical treatment

Where an adolescent has had loss of physical function over a number of months due to pain or if pain is the direct result of an injury or condition (such as CRPS) specialist assessment and possible treatment from an occupational therapist, physiotherapist or other qualified therapists is necessary. Maximising healing and function are necessary before a process of increasing fitness can safely occur. Treatments may involve any of the following.

⊃ Exercises for strengthening targeted muscles to counteract muscle imbalance or weakness and relieve over-worked areas of the body that compensate for the weakness.

⊃ Massage of muscles to release muscle tension and increase circulation or to soften scar tissue.

⊃ Stretches to lengthen muscles that have become tight from disuse.

⊃ Graded desensitisation programme to decrease allodynia.

⊃ Ultrasound to increase healing.

Some of these treatments may be used in conjunction with pharmacological agents or interventions from medical practitioners, such as iontophoresis, cortisone injections or nerve blocks usually performed by an anaesthetist, rheumatologist or orthopaedic surgeon (*see* Chapter 2).

Managing pain during exercise

■ Establish that any pain they may have is not damage or harm!
■ Assess the habits of mind of the adolescent.
■ Every adolescent is different. Work with what you've got!

It is important that the adolescent understands pain physiology (*see* Chapter 1) and pain caused by exercise. If there is enduring underlying belief that pain is harm or damage it is likely that any exercise or fitness programme will be resisted. The prospect of increased movement may trigger fear, anxiety reactions and hypervigilance to pain or body sensations. The mindfulness meditation suggested in Chapter 6, plus a prior commitment to persevering with the task despite these negative thoughts and sensations are necessary. There is no single answer to assisting an adolescent to manage pain as each individual operates differently. Constant reminding that this pain is not harm may be necessary, even repeated out loud for those adolescents experiencing difficulty in holding the idea, or for those who are less adaptable.

Every mind is different!

Habitual ways of dealing with pain may already be apparent at the initial assessment. It is useful to think about this prior to beginning a fitness programme.

Some common habits of mind are apparent in pain management especially in those who are having difficulty.

- Frequent attention to body sensations either as verbal references, or physical actions (scratching, adjusting, touching body parts), or inability to tolerate normal degrees of discomfort indicating a body focus (somatising).
- Lack of awareness of body sensations may be apparent from the adolescent's inability to identify feeling states and sensations in the body such as those accompanying feelings of fear or relaxation. This is characteristic of the over-doer who does not recognise sensations of fatigue. Pain may be the first sign for them.
- Ignoring or avoiding body sensations and 'pushing through' fatigue, pain or discomfort frequently leads to poorly paced activity and frequent, unmanaged pain flare-ups. Although distraction may not be the most useful technique, this is usually the adolescent's preferred option for pain management. It can lead to a spiral of fear avoidance mechanisms.
- Language that is colourful or excessive in describing pain indicates the 'catastrophiser'. This is often a characteristic of adolescents with a vivid imagination. They imaginatively fill in gaps of knowledge with images that exaggerate or misrepresent. Their imaginations can be employed as a positive rather than a negative influence. They can be taught to distract their attention.

Work with what you've got!

Help the ignorers, avoiders or those unaware of sensation to discriminate between the pains, i.e. the original pain and what a stretch feels like. This may require demonstrating with them this experience on a non-painful part of their body. This is part of a process of 'mindfulness' in the body enhanced by relaxation processes, awareness of breath and the ability to look at, rather than away from, sensations.

For less verbal adolescents who find discrimination difficult, start to use words that fit the known differences, i.e. 'pulling and tight' as different from a 'burning or aching' of an injury or 'heaviness' of fatigue. For an adolescent identified as somatising, this focus on sensation is unsuitable, as it encourages focus on the body.

Catastrophisers may be helped with imagery of a cooling, relaxing or healing colour and the substitution of 'overheated' or exaggerated language by words that minimise. 'It's agony' becomes 'It's a bit sore just now.' Talk this through before a process of exercise or exercises begin.

Recognition of unhelpful thoughts with helpful thoughts said out loud (*see* Chapter 6) during the process is useful.

Consciousness of breathing (*see* Chapter 7) is important, as is making sure that the out-breath coincides with the movement if pain increases, i.e. at the end of a stretch – 'making space'. Awareness of breath during movement even, in when simply walking, relaxes, teaches mindfulness and eases tension.

- Taking action increases a belief in ability to cope.
- Increasing self-efficacy decreases pain.

Keeping up fitness: likely barriers

It is worth taking time to work out with the adolescent what the likely barriers to independently keeping or even increasing levels of fitness might be. The final goals identified early on in therapy, such as playing competitive sport, may not be reached on completion of support by the therapist or team. Nevertheless planning a path that allows these goals to be completed is important as part of the process of independence and withdrawal from therapy.

Possible barriers include the following.
- Pain flare-ups in the absence of a flare-up plan (*see* Chapter 6).
- Poor time management, e.g. coinciding with exams.
- Relapse into old habits, e.g. overdoing it or underdoing it, passive coping (not telling others what they need).
- Fitness dependent on external factors, e.g. gym or pool membership, parent transport.
- Inability to maintain discipline.
- Poor planning of transition from home/hospital levels of activity to school/sport activity.

Possible solutions
- Discuss transition from the support phase using lower-level goals (such as walking for half an hour) in order to set new goals. Choose recording of practice using charts or graphs or whatever form has been successful.

If the goal is to play competitive basketball/netball, add into the goal numbers of jumps or free play using jumps and ball for 15 minutes. Once the adolescent reaches this level of ability, they are usually able to take the next steps independently.

⊃ In preparing for a goal (shopping, return to school, etc.) make sure that the number of preparation practices for the activity matches the real-life task. Walking for 15 minutes around the house may not be equal to walking around the school yard plus catching a bus home. Advice to increase the amount of home walking practice before returning to school and finding an alternative to a bus journey will ensure a more successful outcome.

⊃ Set up networks of support at school to assist in advocating on the adolescent's behalf.

⊃ Ask the adolescent to commit to making regular follow-up telephone calls to you during the transition to independence time.

⊃ Make sure that activities are achievable without dependence on others.

⊃ Hydrotherapy four times a week but only available in one season may be substituted with one yoga class, one 40-minute walk on the weekend, one physical education class at school and one bike ride with the family.

Case study: Hannah

Hannah was a 16-year-old high school student. Hannah was the only child in a household comprising her single-parent mother and her grandmother. Despite the two jobs worked by the mother, finances were tight.

Hannah had injured her left shoulder in an incident during army cadet training one year prior to her presentation at a pain-management clinic. She reported extreme pain on movement and range of movement limited to a few degrees in all directions. She walked holding her left arm immobile across her front.

The incident in the course of which the injury had occurred had been reported to the mental health authority under the mandatory reporting required for sexual abuse. Following the reporting, Hannah had refused treatment or counselling and continued her attendance at cadets despite the ongoing presence of the perpetrator of the abuse. When asked about the event she stated that she believed in toughing out any emotional difficulties, identifying herself with her deceased grandfather who had been a soldier and a heroic member of the Dutch resistance during World War II. The grandmother, who frequently likened her granddaughter to her 'stubborn' husband, endorsed this identification. Hannah's grandmother and mother felt unable to influence Hannah's 'stubbornness'.

Hannah refused to limit any of her activities despite her considerable limitation, continuing to work at the local take-away restaurant twice a week and attending cadets also twice a week. She had a ranking at cadets that required her to train juniors, which she took very seriously, refusing to 'let them down' at parades and events. Her only concession was not to participate in parades that required marching.

Rehabilitation on her shoulder did not progress for one year as Hannah also refused to concede any of her activities for attendance at her physiotherapy outpatient appointments. Her mother and grandmother seemed unable to make her attend, appointments were repeatedly cancelled or cut short because of her activities, which she felt were of greater importance. She constantly found excuses saying she had to work as she had to save money for herself to get into military college, she couldn't let other recruits down, etc.

Finally the team presented to Hannah and her mother the likely scenario for Hannah her if she continued to evade appointments and rehabilitation. Hannah decided that she would submit to an intense period of rehabilitation as an in-patient. She was to receive twice-daily physiotherapy and twice-daily occupational therapy including pain-management techniques. She continued to refuse psychological help.

In the first week of therapy, Hannah was defensive and prickly in her responses to learning self-management techniques, particularly the relaxation techniques, often wanting to appear as though she already knew what to do. Hannah's main strategy for pain management that she had identified was distraction and avoidance. Discussion around these techniques lead to an understanding that avoidance had not served her well as her physical status had not changed and it was likely to be maintaining a fear of movement. Hannah began to learn to look at the pain rather than avoid it and to apply breathing techniques to manage it while doing her physiotherapy exercises, gradually increasing her movements (*see* Chapter 6 for more details).

By the end of her in-patient stay, her range of movement had increased and she felt she was coping with her pain. She was compliant and non-combative with therapists, smiling and joking in sessions. At the point of returning home, she accepted that she had to pace herself rather than ignoring her body messages as she had in the past. She accepted that she should limit her work hours and modify her duties at work. She set goals in the Canadian Occupational Performance Measure that included carrying her backpack weighing 8 kilograms for 6 minutes and to march with her arm in extension for 2 minutes. On her return home, she paced herself with her pack, first carrying her schoolbag with a 1-kilogram book for 6 minutes – then increasing this weight by half a kilogram at a time sustaining the increase daily for one week before increasing the weight again. In this way she was able to reach her goal over several months of paced, increased activity.

Comment

Hannah's early progress had been impeded by a number of factors. Her desire not to accept counselling for what had clearly been a major trauma was respected by the team but was nevertheless likely to have contributed to her habitual avoidance behaviour. This avoidance had, in turn, impeded her ability to change or move forward. The family stories that likened the 16-year-old girl to a war hero endorsed behaviour that was dysfunctional and led to a disempowering of parental authority. Rehabilitation progressed only when the pain clinic team assumed this authority.

However, Hannah's reputation as a self-manager and disciplinarian eventually served her well in her determination to assume responsibility to pace herself in order to achieve her physical goals.

References

1 Walter AS, Williamson GMK. The role of activity restriction in the association between pain and depression: a study of paediatric patients with chronic pain. *Children's Health Care.* 1999; **28**(1): 33–50.

2 Bandura A. *Self-efficacy: the exercise of control.* New York: WH Freeman; 1997.

3 Eldridge B, Galea M, McCoy A, *et al.* Uptime normative values in children aged 8–15 years. *Dev Med Child Neurol.* 2003; **45**: 189–93.

4 Birkholtz M, Aylwin L, Harma RM. Activity pacing in chronic pain management: one aim but which method? Part one: Introduction and literature review. *British Journal of Occupational Therapy.* 2004; **67**(10): 447–52.

CHAPTER 10

Returning to school

WHAT INFLUENCES A SUCCESSFUL PLAN?

CHAPTER SUMMARY

This chapter is designed to present a possible process that will assist in returning the adolescent to school. An assessment process that identifies issues likely to impact on return to school is outlined in questions, with a discussion on school refusal. Setting goals with the adolescent and identifying the needs and problems of schools are addressed, as are the principal requirements for a graduated return-to-school plan. The many psychosocial issues that are associated with this process are identified. Common concerns from the adolescent's perspective are addressed. Finally, a process is outlined with a suggested informal contract between all parties concerned.

Background

The process suggested here will always need to be tailored to the individual adolescent's particularities. Timing may be longer or shorter according to progress made in other areas including fitness, counselling or skills in managing pain or sleep. This chapter is not designed to look at these 'non-school' issues as they have been addressed in other chapters. However, many issues raised in the earlier chapters will need to have been addressed as their outcome will influence a return-to-school programme. There is little information about how schools deal with adolescents with persistent pain; however, this chapter will also address the needs of schools as identified in the literature.[1]

There is a paucity of research beyond the effect of persistent pain on school attendance. Persistent pain from a wide range of chronic illnesses significantly affects school attendance, with headaches, abdominal pain and musculoskeletal pain being the most common.[2,3] What is less known empirically is the relationship of persistent pain to academic performance, academic competence and classroom behaviour. Some of these relationships are observable clinically, with suggestion of support in the literature.[4,5,6] Some of these issues are addressed in the following chapter.

Assessment

A thorough biopsychosocial assessment is required to identify all issues that may be relevant to school life. This will need to include issues addressed in earlier chapters – such as earlier fitness, pain coping, separation difficulties, family functioning, etc. The following is a list of areas directly pertaining to school that are relevant to explore as appropriate. (*See* Chapter 1.)

➲ What school does the adolescent go to?
➲ What year are they in?
➲ Have they been to other schools in the past? When?
➲ What were the reasons for change?
➲ Do they like school?
➲ What do they like/not like about school?
➲ What are their major difficulties at school?
➲ What are their friendships?
➲ Have they been bullied?
➲ If so, when and what happened at that time?
➲ How much school has been missed? Why?
➲ Do they currently achieve a full day at school?
➲ If not, what is the process of deciding to not go, or leave early?
➲ In what way does pain interfere?
➲ Are they able to keep up with any friends?
➲ How are they going academically in relations to their peers?
➲ How do they get to and from school and how long does it take?
➲ Whom would they prefer to nominate as their contact person?

Once the above information has been gathered, it may become apparent that there is a history of school-attendance issues either in the adolescent's past, prior to pain, or that school attendance has been an issue for other siblings. It is important to correctly diagnose the problem that prevents the child attending school. It is often difficult to make a clear distinction between school refusal or school phobia and the management of pain at school, as pain can be a somatic complaint that is associated with school phobia and which successfully maintains the status quo of absenteeism. The treatment for both is the same, i.e. a supported, graduated return to school with counselling to manage associated conditions (such as anxiety).

School refusal and phobias

An indicator of pain as a somatic complaint which successfully maintains absenteeism is the timing of pain flare-ups at the beginning of a new school term, or on Sunday evenings just prior to the school week. Parents who are critical of the school and who believe unquestioningly their adolescent's reasons, may not see this pattern.

Several attempts at classification of school phobia (sometimes called school refusal) have been made.[7] Factors identified as significant in this condition are: patterns of family interactions, anxiety in the adolescent, anxiety in the mother, a dependent mother–child relationship, overindulgent or controlling parenting style, academic difficulties, borderline intelligence, schizophrenia or other adolescent crisis.[8] As can be seen in previous chapters, many of these factors impact on adolescents with persistent pain who present for treatment.

Phobias are described as a maladaptive avoidance response maintained by reduction of fear (i.e. of school or of leaving home), the fear reducing when the adolescent returns home to the parent who reinforces the avoidant behaviour of allowing them to stay at home.[9]

The treatment for school phobias is a supported, graduated return to school. Pharmacological agents may be necessary to assist in the initial management of somatic symptomatology.

School attendance as a goal

It is possible also for a return to school to be proposed and for it to proceed with the simplest of interventions such as a session with parents, a letter or phone call to the school. This is only likely with a strong history of school attendance prior to the pain event, a clearly identified goal of return to school, a co-operative school and parent, and an appropriate level of fitness.

Working out strategies for returning to school can be a shared process with a willing adolescent when there is a clear goal identified by the adolescent arising from preliminary values-based work (*see* Chapter 5).

There are many reasons that most adolescents want to go to school. They like to be with friends and they get increased self-esteem from positive feedback from achievements. It is also normal for peer-group approval to be increasingly more important than approval from their parents. It is always significant if return to school is not one of the goals chosen in the initial goal-setting process. The goal-setting process may be the first place where this 'yellow flag' becomes apparent. The adolescent or parent may simply forget to mention it. It is important to consider why this might be. There are no rules and each adolescent and family will be unique. Values-based work may reveal a discrepancy between the adolescent's and the parents' values.

What the school needs

Schools, like parents, want to know how to deal with an adolescent presenting with persistent pain.

The same questions that arise for parents, also arise for teachers:

⊃ Is ongoing pain a sign of ongoing damage?
⊃ What is the diagnosis?
⊃ How do I get reliable information?
⊃ What can I do that is helpful?
⊃ How much can I expect the adolescent to do when they have pain?
⊃ Is the pain real?

A prior medical assessment and diagnosis are necessary so that an explanation can be made to teachers. A simple explanation of basic pain physiology will usually allay questions of whether the pain is real (*see* Chapter 1). It will also explain the relationship of pain and stress and other psychological issues. Informing the school that physical guidelines will be recommended is reassuring and prevents conflict between the adolescent, the family and school. Being available for contact by teachers is helpful, as is explaining the aims of the return-to-school programme. Such an explanation can change attitudes, or dampen conflict and ill-feeling that may have arisen.

The assessment format and case formulation in Chapter 1 should provide basic information required to construct a return-to-school programme – in particular to diagnose the cause of school absenteeism which may be influenced by combinations of a number of things, i.e. avoidant behaviours as in a phobia, poor sleep, pain or poor fitness, peer relationship problems, anxiety or depression, or academic difficulties.

A graduated return-to-school plan

In formulating a graduated return-to-school plan, some principles need to be observed.

⊃ If stamina or endurance is an issue (this can be physical endurance or even endurance of social interaction for a child with social anxiety), the principles of pacing are required. The agreed time of graduated exposure to the goals (such as sitting or walking) or to the socialising needs to be such that it is sustainable for several days or even weeks before a new or extended time is set. (*See* 'Pacing' in Chapter 9.) Devise conservative goals since an inability to sustain the plan leads to disappointment and confirms the chronicity of the problem in the adolescent's mind.

- ⊃ The times of arrival and departure, once agreed, must be non-negotiable. The initial timetable is likely to require the input of the adolescent as it will entail timetabling core subjects and estimation of tolerances. If the main cause of school refusal is phobia or poor sleep patterns, the time of arrival should be by the first school period. It is important that the times of arrival and departure are adhered to. If times start to blur, then it becomes apparent that the decision to come and go are being made by the adolescent based on how they *feel* that day. There may also be a lack of will on the part of the parent. Adolescents who accept negative feelings as the driver of whether to attend school or not are likely to also feel uncertain and insecure. It is ultimately disempowering as feelings (including the feeling of pain!) become the boss and the adolescent once again feels out of control (this is dealt with in more detail in Chapter 5). Values-based work and mindfulness training will support the adolescent's commitment to continue despite having negative feelings at the decision time.
- ⊃ Poor sleep needs to have been addressed (*see* Chapter 4).
- ⊃ Conditions for unwellness (e.g. viruses) need to be made explicit. (That is, illness sufficient to warrant a visit to the local general practitioner who understands the issues. This may require contact with the general practitioner to alert her/him to the issues.)
- ⊃ Timeliness must be adhered to. It is part of the socialising process in Western society; it is required for appointments, for school, for exams and for work. Ultimately it is an expectation of adulthood and is part of the learning that occurs in adolescents, i.e. the gradual assumption of responsibility – in this case, responsibility for being on time.
- ⊃ Parents need to understand their role. This may mean helping them to learn parenting skill, to insist on a bedtime regime, timeliness in the morning, or making staying at home less attractive and rewarding, etc.

Common difficulties expressed by adolescents with persistent pain and needing to return to school after some absence are:
- ⊃ What will I do when I get pain?
- ⊃ How will my energy last the day? What if I can't cope?
- ⊃ How will I be able to concentrate with the pain?
- ⊃ Am I able to keep up with the class? If not, how will I catch up with schoolwork?
- ⊃ How will I get from place to place?
- ⊃ What will I be able to do in physical education classes?
- ⊃ What will I say to my school mates? Will my friends still like me if I can't share the same sports and social activities?

Pain can become a means of avoiding other more longstanding or seemingly insoluble problems for an adolescent. It can be a way of 'saving face'. Teaching pain-management skills will not produce a return to school if the non-attendance at school is a more positive experience than attendance at school, i.e. reinforced with other rewards such as staying at grandma's house or watching TV at home.

⊶ 'Yellow flags'

These may alert the therapist or team to the need for further investigation and management.

- **An injury at school** that could be interpreted as being the result of the school's negligence. This requires a frank discussion regarding the likelihood of litigation. Litigation significantly changes the working relationship with the school and the expectancy of a positive outcome from therapy.
- **An increase in pain on Sunday evenings** or at the beginning of the school term.
  This warrants investigation into the source of the negative experience anticipated by the adolescent (bullying, failure, etc.) and the reinforcers for the avoidant behaviour.
- **A history of poor school attendance.** (See below.)
- Identifiable **separation difficulties** at the beginning of kindergarten or the first year of school.
  This indicates the need for counselling with the mother.
- **A history of poor social relationships** in school.
  Assessment by a psychologist and counselling for the adolescent, preferably locally where access to support can be ongoing can help.
- **Bullying** of a longstanding nature, either present or past.
- Signs of **academic struggle**.
  A psychological assessment of cognitive function, e.g. WISC, may clarify learning needs. This should be followed by parent counselling on appropriate school choices.

Likely issues associated with 'yellow flags'

History of poor school attendance

This may be related to a parent who:
- is unable to insist on a routine, thereby having allowed many absences from school in the past and an unspoken acceptance of this
- is unable to face any disagreement with their child, fearing alienating their child, i.e. the child is the one with the power to make the decision
- fears that their child may be ill when they are not
- enjoys the company of their child during the day
- has reinforced avoidant coping with the withdrawal of the adolescent to the comfort at home rather than learned outward coping

⊃ has past history of difficulty separating and allowing new independence

⊃ has no other interests in their life, fearing loneliness or boredom without their 'best friend' child resulting in a 'parentified' child who feels responsible for them and assumes the parental role

⊃ who has undiagnosed learning difficulty.

Transition stage

The transition from primary school to secondary school or starting at a new school may be problematic. The adolescent:

⊃ may not have made new friendships or has difficulty where friendship groups are already established

⊃ may fear independence or failure. Expectations placed on the adolescent for academic success can be made by the adolescent with perfectionist tendencies, by the parents or by the school. The parents may have specifically chosen the school for that purpose and it may not match the adolescent's inclinations

⊃ may be perceived as a 'gifted' child by parents who set the child apart socially from peers or cause performance anxiety in their child

⊃ does not make independent decisions because parents have been very involved in the child's early schooling

⊃ may find themselves in a school being the less 'brilliant' younger child following a highly successful 'brilliant' older sibling.

Case study: Miriam

Another father employed within the education department as a consultant had instigated enrichment classes that his 'gifted' daughter attended. He was ambitious for his gifted child. She was already a year ahead of her age group, and was having difficulty coping socially as she was seen as a 'geek' by her peers! Her pain had started with an incident at school, when she had a fall while lifting a rowing scull, sustaining a soft-tissue injury of her wrist. She recalled that when she fell, her team mates were laughing at her.

Her father and teacher mother stated quite clearly that they did not want their daughter to be a teacher as this was beneath her and that she was to go to university to become a doctor. At the point of referral, their daughter had developed extreme, unmanageable pain and tremor in her writing hand, despite investigations revealing no sign of damage. It was observed that her tremor disappeared at inconsistent times. Her pain diminished when she stayed at home but increased again on Sunday evenings and at the end of holidays. Her parents were extremely agitated and anxious, pressuring their daughter and the treating team to 'cure' their daughter so that she could sit her exams. They were angry and devastated when she was unable to sit the exams that would have allowed her to attend university a year ahead of normal year level. Her parents withdrew her from treatment, preferring to seek a cure for what they felt was an undiscovered medical condition.

Unrecognised learning difficulties

Difficulties may be unrecognised because:
⊃ the parents or school are uninterested
⊃ bad behaviour by the adolescent masks the difficulty
⊃ parents are in denial of the difficulty.

Case study: Brigit

Brigit, aged 14 years, had unmanageable pain in her knee following patella instability. She had had successful physiotherapy to strengthen the knee but continued to report that the patella slipped, causing extreme pain, especially at school. She had stopped her favourite sporting activity of swimming and had stayed at home to manage her pain and had withdrawn from social activity. Brigit reported that teachers did not like her because she had 'a big mouth' and sometimes challenged her teachers. Her mother reported that she had no trouble academically but that she and her daughter were seen as trouble makers.

Contact with the school revealed that Brigit was disruptive, inattentive and distracting to others in class. Teachers did not report any academic difficulty. A Wechsler IQ test showed considerable discrepancy between the child's performance and her academic level of placement at school. The girl was unable to understand her class work and became disruptive, causing teachers to focus on behaviour rather than on academic performance. Her difficulties were not acknowledged by her or her parents as they had unrealistic vocational goals, having nominated a career in physiotherapy. Brigit learned to acknowledge that her pain was exacerbated by stress which had several sources, one of which was her issues at school. A second was that, following her early experiences, she greatly feared displacement of her patella. She believed there was still physical damage associated with her pain. A follow-up MRI was sufficient to prove to her that there was no continuing damage. She recommended swimming, the school was alerted to her learning difficulties and she was given extra assistance in her areas of need. She recommended full-time school.

School culture

Parents may not be aware of the needs of their child and may choose a school that matches their values and ambitions rather than their child's. The school chosen may:

⊃ have poor tolerance of individual needs or difference
⊃ have a mismatch of values, e.g. a sporty, macho, single-sex boys' school for a boy interested in singing and drama or academia
⊃ be ill-equipped and understaffed
⊃ have a culture of not responding to parents' or adolescent's requests
⊃ have no policy to manage bullying.

Case study: Tony

Tony was a physically immature boy of 13 years of age, who was smaller than his more physically boisterous, athletic younger brother. He presented initially with complex regional pain of his knee, having injured himself in a rough game with his brother. He was attending his first year of secondary school in an all-boys school. The school was reputed to focus on sport and had a strong physically 'macho' culture in the playground and sports field.

Tony had had several attempts to return to school only to fail because of re-injury of the knee and a new injury to his shoulder. This occurred either at home with his brother or in the playground at school. Tony reported that it was difficult to make friends because he was unable to play the sports and games that underpinned the prevailing social culture of the school. Tony's parents insisted he stay at this school because of the religious affinity and because there was the financial advantage of having two boys at the same school. Initially, Tony was on crutches, then was restricted by his ability to walk any distance. He had difficulty getting from one classroom to another on time and had problems persuading the school that he required exemption from sporting activities.

Communication with the school was difficult as his co-ordinator was initially unobtainable, as was his teacher. Finally, when telephone contact with the school was made, it appeared that no concessions were made for him, with some teachers keeping him in for late arrival to class. The general belief was that Tony was making up his pain and injuries because they recurred frequently, they went on for so long and because he complained so much. A school visit was arranged to meet the co-ordinator together with Tony's mother, in order to explain his condition and the return-to-school programme. However, no further understanding or concessions for Tony resulted from the meeting, confirming what his mother had reported.

The school this young boy was required to attend was unsuitable for him. The school was uncommunicative and inflexible, with a culture that did not embrace difference and, despite the fact that the school was on a considerable slope with hills and steps between classrooms, no concessions were ever made for Tony. The unspoken school culture did not allow Tony to feel able to withdraw to practise his relaxation strategies and it was impossible for him to pace himself according to his abilities. Underlying Tony's return-to-school problems was a more fundamental family disagreement between his parents as to the suitability of the school. His father supported the 'macho' culture and felt it was the best place for Tony as it would encourage him to be tougher and more physical. The parents were unwilling to accept counselling to resolve this and Tony continued to re-present at other clinics within the hospital.

Over-sympathetic teachers
- The teacher may have personal experience of pain or other disability and inappropriately identify with the adolescent.
- The teacher may see themselves as 'rescuing' the adolescent and may treat the adolescent as special, unnecessarily maintaining physical dependence, social separation or emotional immaturity.

Case study: Susie

Susie was a pretty 12-year-old girl with a history of recurrent abdominal pain of unknown aetiology and whose longstanding history of poor school attendance was worsened by over-sympathetic teachers. Following assessment, Susie was found to have a great need to please, with a history of staying in with the teacher during recess to help her, and generally being the teacher's pet. Her parents were both generally anxious people who felt that Susie had an undiagnosed condition yet to be found.

Susie's teacher had become a friend of the family following her offer of help. The teacher had been going to Susie's house after school hours and had been home-tutoring her. The teacher herself experienced persistent pain and felt that she understood Susie's pain. Susie was quite able to keep up with school work for several terms in this way, having no difficulty in concentration or physical stamina. The parents were counselled on pain physiology, the diagnosis and its relationship to anxiety, stress and pain. They were advised of helpful behavioural strategies for their daughter and accepted ongoing counselling. Susie also required ongoing counselling to deal with her social anxiety. These changes underpinned the general change that allowed a return to school; however, it was also required that the teacher should understand what she needed to do to be helpful for Susie.

Poor understanding or communication between teachers
- Teachers may not understand the child's need for rest breaks, implying disbelief and that the adolescent is 'faking' the pain.

⊃ Some physical education teachers believe the 'no pain no gain!' slogan and that pain is a barrier that needs to be 'broken through'.

⊃ Teachers may not provide catch-up homework for absences, causing anxiety and feelings of hopelessness.

Physical barriers of school layout

⊃ Placement of lockers may be at the wrong height, or where student will be knocked, or too far away.

⊃ The distance between classrooms, and classrooms being upstairs may extend the adolescent's physical endurance beyond its current limit.

⊃ Physical placement of classrooms rather than core subjects may dictate what subjects can or cannot be attended, causing stress for the adolescent.

Poor advocacy for the adolescent

⊃ School can be large and sometimes chaotic, particularly in the yard during breaks. This can be especially so for socially phobic, Asperger's syndrome adolescents or those with CRPS and sensitivity to knocks and bumps.

⊃ Quiet children may not be heard.

⊃ Parents may be unwilling or unable to advocate for their child.

⊃ Adolescent or parents may have fallen foul of a particular co-ordinator.

⊃ The school may be poorly resourced and unable to co-ordinate a special programme or to adapt classrooms.

⊃ Internal political turmoil may inhibit the school's ability to manage an individual child's need.

⊃ There may be an unrealistic expectation that the child will co-ordinate homework with teachers, leaving the unassertive adolescent feeling powerless. Teachers may not co-ordinate the homework load or timetable among themselves, thereby causing stress for the adolescent with high academic expectations.

Explaining to peer group

Peer relationships are paramount in adolescence: what friends or peers think and say is more important than most things. Adolescents may:

⊃ feel that their peers will be curious and nosey or will tease them

⊃ fear being different and 'uncool'

⊃ worry that their peer group has forgotten them after a long absence

⊃ feel that no visible sign of injury might lead to disbelief amongst peers.

A process for return to school

Do a thorough initial assessment and case formulation (refer to Chapter 1).

⊃ Phone the school and ask to speak to the person likely to know this student the best. It may be the co-ordinator, the form teacher, the pastoral carer or the counsellor. Ask for their perception of the adolescent's social interaction, academic performance any other incidents of significance. Schools, like parents, want to know what to do when pain occurs. They want to know what helpful, appropriate action is. It is important to let them know that strategies will be set up to which all parties agree.

⊃ Formulate for yourself the likely difficulties. Only some of these may be identified or understood by the adolescent and their family. Having an hypothesis allows the possibility of testing it out in the application of the return-to-school programme. For instance, suggesting psychological testing can be a shock or even a threat for some parents. They may not have considered that their child has any difficulties (such as low-level Asperger's or learning difficulties.) It may challenge their sense of themselves as attentive or understanding parents. It may also challenge their dreams for their child.

⊃ Work with the child, address their concerns and problem-solve with their co-operation. If bullying has been a problem consult the school about the school policy. Go over this with the child and make sure that they have an appropriate contact person that they trust at the school. A longstanding history of problems with bullying may need to be dealt with by means of ongoing psychological counselling.

Common concerns of the adolescent

'What will I do when I get pain?'

Accept the child's pain as a reality. How to deal with the pain will be upper-most in the adolescent's mind. (Refer to Chapter 7 on relaxation, distraction and mindfulness and to Chapter 6 on what to do with the pain.) From their perspective, this is the first and most important barrier to overcome. Give the adolescent choices of where to do relaxation. Some will be willing to learn to apply it in the classroom while for others it needs to be very private and without their peers knowing. Being different can be the worst imaginable thing for some adolescents. Be adaptable in recommendations so that they are workable for them. The results of these negotiations form the basis of the 'contract' for a return to school. At times it may be appropriate to involve parents in strategies for accepting a routine and agreeing not to fetch their child outside of the agreed timetable.

'How will my energy last the day? What if I can't cope?'

In respect of the physical goals and measured tolerances, work with a map of the school and estimated distances between core-subject classrooms to work out optimum attendance times. This can then be presented to the school with a request for either academic support or suggestions for class arrangements.

Discuss rest/relaxation breaks to be taken at school instead of the adolescent going home to rest. It is possible to mock up the pacing required before the start of school term. Make sure there are rewards for coping, negotiated preferably with the adolescent first or with the parent. The reward does not need to be a bought material object, it may be time spent with a favourite person, or an event.

Poor sleep is often a reason for increased pain, late arrival at school and poor concentration. (*See* Chapter 4 for detailed sleep management plan.)

'How will I be able to concentrate with the pain?'

Acknowledge that pain is a distraction and remind the adolescent of the physiology of distraction and the nature of pain as alarm. Teach mindfulness and refocusing. Use flash cards that are to be kept at school, e.g. 'This pain is not harm,' 'Getting back to my work is a way of coping,' 'It's natural that pain will interrupt.' Revisit the process of learning relaxation using it as a model: accept that the mind wanders without getting upset; it is normal for pain to interrupt, notice it, but bring attention back and congratulate yourself whenever you manage to do this. Do not let the adolescent say, 'I *tried* that' as this contains implied failure 'I tried . . . (but failed!).' *Any* action taken is a measure of success and ability.

'Am I able to keep up with the class? If not, how will I catch up with schoolwork?'

Finding an advocate or co-ordinator within the school whom the adolescent finds approachable can be helpful. The ability to independently seek help may be part of the adolescent's learning process, and this seeking of help may be best done without the parent's intervention and with the therapist or counsellor's support. Again each student and school is different and each needs to be assessed for their situation at the time.

'How will I get from place to place?'

If the physical layout of the school is a problem, get a map of the school and the classrooms, and a copy of the timetable. Identify the classrooms for the core subjects and estimate the approximate distance between classrooms, either in time taken or even in number of steps required between classrooms. These distances and frequency of walking or stair climbing become the detail of the goals (*see* Chapter 5). Modification of the number of classes attended may be necessary, depending on the current level of fitness. Timetable modification plus minimising distance travelled to lockers or playground may be part of the discussions with the school. The adolescent or school may have preferred solutions but remember, it will not work if the adolescent does not see it as workable for them.

'What will I be able to do in physical education classes?'

Suggest a letter that the adolescent and parent has a copy of, that clearly states the student's current physical capacities and limitations, specifically covering the areas of concern identified by the adolescent. This may include such issues as distance to the sports field, as well as rest breaks, etc.

'What will I say to my school mates? Will my friends still like me if I can't share the same sports and social activities?'

Explaining the existence of pain without apparent injury can be difficult. Role-playing what to say can be very helpful. Scripting and rehearsing stock phrases that the adolescent feels comfortable saying and that satisfy curiosity but prevent further enquiry may be helpful. Working out with the adolescent, perhaps by listing why friends might still like them, or listing other activities they can share, can be reassuring.

Case study: Bernie

(*See* Chapter 5 for more general background details of this case.)

Bernie was an adolescent boy of 13 years diagnosed with CRPS. He had a history of poor attendance at primary school. In the past, his mother had allowed him to stay home from school and to accompany her to her workplace where she would help him with his school work.

Bernie had been absent for two terms of his first year of high school following a few months' attendance. He felt insecure about his friendships, as he had had only a short time at the new school before he developed knee pain that was accompanied by convulsive shaking of the leg. He stated at his initial meeting that he had never liked school but that for the first time he liked his new school and wanted to attend regularly. In his early therapy sessions, he learnt what activity exacerbated his knee pain and he learned strategies to manage activity and the pain. He had also accepted during the process of his visits that his shakes followed by the spasms were often associated with generalised anxiety and his attention to 'weird' sensations. At one point, he developed pain in his hand, which then became immobilised. He learned strategies to manage this by attending and recording whenever it moved (*see* Chapter 5, on goals). With the occupational therapist, he was taught strategies to focus on his breathing when he felt 'weird', to use different language and to accept his body sensations. Psychological counselling helped him identify feelings of anxiety that were associated with pain flare-ups. He had regular physiotherapy to increase function until he was able to manage a full day at school.

A return-to-school programme was constructed, in which the physical layout, walking distances and his current mobility levels were matched with the key subject classes he needed to attend. His year co-ordinator organised support and a catch-up programme in conjunction with his teachers. However, one of his main obstacles was what to say on his return to school. Bernie knew his peers would be curious and he did not want to say the same thing over and over to every person who asked him; he did not want them being overly interested and he was fearful of having a bout of the shaking in front of his peers. Bernie rehearsed options of what he would feel comfortable saying, and he chose to address his whole class on the first day of his return to school. He gave a brief but general description of what had happened with a reference to the pain system continuing to fire off even after the original injury had mended. He said that he was getting better and that it was better not to ask him about it, as it was not helpful. If his knee started to jump, to ignore it because he could manage it himself. When he was contacted 18 months later, he had had no occurrences of spasms, he had remained at school full time and had returned to playing basketball.

An informal 'contract' example

The adolescent agrees to the following:

⊃ To attend school at the times nominated in the prepared timetable. The time at which they go home should be a set time and should not be dependent on pain level or the adolescent's desire to go home

⊃ To manage the prevention of flare-ups by regular relaxation at recess and in spare periods even when no pain is evident

⊃ To manage any increase in pain by taking action early, i.e. by going to a sickbay (library, empty classroom, etc.) where they will practise the strategies agreed upon (relaxation, visualisation, stretches, etc.). If they lie down when they go home, they can lie down in sickbay. If pain persists they may perhaps do this for a set period of time

⊃ On the first day to address the class (or friends) to explain what has happened

⊃ To contact therapist by phone in the first week/fortnight for a progress report

⊃ To contact the school counsellor on an as-needs basis regarding exam stress

⊃ To accept that any reward is a temporary encouragement rather than a permanent fixture of school attendance.

The parent agrees to the following:

⊃ To attend school only at the prescribed times and not to respond to phone calls from the adolescent

⊃ Not to ask the child if they have pain or if they do not feel well enough to go to school

⊃ That if unwellness is reported, then illness confirmation is required from the family doctor or by fever, etc. (Doctor to have a copy of this contract and accompanying letter, with parents' and adolescent's agreement.)

⊃ That if pain is reported, then parent is to request adolescent to practise pain-management strategies before going to school

⊃ To supply the 'reward' agreed upon with their child for a number of successful days attendance at school. Examples of rewards include special outings, new clothing or music. (The reward is not necessarily ongoing.)

The school agrees to the following:

⊃ To supply extra work as required
⊃ To make some physical changes, e.g. classroom availability, making a lift available, changing locker arrangements, allowing longer exam time
⊃ That the school nurse will allow the adolescent to attend sickbay according to the plan, and to practise the agreed strategies. (Nurse to have a copy of the contract with a letter if required.)
⊃ To note times of sickbay attendance for recording of agreed goal of decreasing time out of classes. (Patterns of sickbay attendance may also show avoidance of a particular subject or source of anxiety, e.g. maths class or a shouting teacher. It may also reveal poor pacing or causes of pain exacerbation.)

The pain therapist agrees to the following:

⊃ To maintain contact with the adolescent and family by phone in the first week and then as required
⊃ To call back if adolescent or parent calls
⊃ To maintain contact with school as required.

Case study: Mathew

Mathew, 12 years of age, presented with unmanageable headache that was accompanied by bouts of a few seconds of temporary fainting or blacking out. He had one of these bouts in the initial interview. The parents were concerned that there was some organic cause for the events. They were already aware that their son was 'different', having unusual interests, different from those of other boys. He was musically gifted, having been taught by his mother; he had poor social skills, his only friend being a disabled boy from an older class that he talked to on the phone; and he was physically clumsy. Mathew developed his headache early in his school year. At that time he had been bullied by a bigger boy in his class. This boy also bullied others in the class but Mathew felt particularly vulnerable. He had told the teacher but although the teacher had given the bully a talking to, Mathew remained intimidated especially as the bullying occurred when the teacher was not within view and after a while the teacher failed to respond to Mathew's request for help. None of this was revealed at the initial assessment, as his parents were primarily concerned that there was an organic cause for Mathew's headache. His headache was so extreme that he no longer attended school and was unable to play the piano, which he had previously played at a very high level (he could remember and play whole Bach sonatas).

Over a period of weeks in therapy, Mathew learned pain-management strategies for his headache, he was able to talk about his problem at school, and he understood that when he had felt things were out of control, he had literally taken 'time out' by blacking out. His parents accepted the non-organic basis for his headache and blackouts. A lengthy negotiated plan was put in place that Mathew felt able to execute in his classroom. The main thrust of his therapy was to allow Mathew to feel in charge. His return-to-school plan included details about how close the bully was allowed to get to him before the teacher would be required to respond. It had been necessary to engage the co-ordinator in the process in order to get the classroom teacher – who had been largely unresponsive – to actively respond to Mathew's needs. Mathew's ability to endure time in the classroom was affected by other factors than the presence of the bully. He found social interactions difficult and tiring and he found it difficult to tolerate noise. As part of his graduated return he was allowed to go to the quiet place at the back of the room and use the headphones as required. For many weeks he was only able to attend for an hour. This increased to an hour and a half. Over a period of months, Mathew's time in the classroom increased. He used the quiet area as needed, rather than blacking out or going home. His parents were counselled on the possibility of Asperger's syndrome. They chose to look for appropriate ongoing help for Mathew's future schooling needs as he entered high school.

References

1 Logan DE, Curran MS. Adolescent chronic pain problems in the school setting: exploring the experiences and beliefs of selected school personnel through focus group methodology. *J Adolesc Health.* 2005; **37**: 281–8.
2 Perquin CW, Hazebroek-Kampschreur AAJM, Hunfeld JAM, *et al.* Pain in children and adolescents: a common experience. *Pain.* 2000; **87**: 51–8.
3 Kristjansdottir G. Prevalence of pain combinations and overall pain: a study of headache, stomach pain and back pain among schoolchildren. *Scand J Soc Med.* 1997; **25**: 58–63.
4 Palermo TM. Impact of recurrent and chronic pain on child and family daily functioning: a critical review of the literature. *J Dev Behav Ped.* 2000; **21**: 58–69.
5 Tsao JC, Glover DA, Bursch B, *et al.* Laboratory pain reactivity and gender: relationship to school nurse visits and school absences. *J Dev Behav Ped.* 2002; **23**: 217–24.
6 Walker LS, Claar RL, Garber J. Social consequences of children's pain: when do they encourage symptom maintenance? *J Pediatr Child Psychol.* 2002; **7**: 689–98.
7 De Sousa A, de Sousa DA. School phobia. *Child Psychiatry Q.* 1980; **13**(4): 98–103.
8 Torma S, Halsti A. Factors contributing to school phobia and truancy. *Psychiatria Fennica.* 1975; **6**: 209–20.
9 Ross AO. Behaviour therapy. In: Quay HC, Werry JS, editors. *Psychopathological Disorders of Childhood*, 3rd ed. New York: Wiley; 1986.

Glossary

Anxiety sensitivity refers to the fear of anxiety-related sensations that are interpreted as having potentially harmful somatic, psychological or social consequences and hence give rise to significant anxiety (Taylor, 1995).

Allodynia is pain due to a stimulus which does not normally provoke pain, e.g. touch is felt as pain.

Analgesia is the absence of pain in response to stimulation which would normally be painful.

Beliefs are assumptions about reality which serve as a perceptual lens, or a 'set' through which events are interpreted (Lazarus and Folkman, 1984).

Catastrophising is expecting or worrying about major negative consequences from a situation, even one of minor importance.

Conversion disorder is a diagnostic category of DSM 1V with the emphasis on alteration or loss of functioning of an organ or body system.

Central pain is pain initiated or caused by a primary lesion or dysfunction in the central nervous system.

Coping is constantly changing cognitive and behavioural efforts to manage specific external and/or internal demands that are appraised as taxing or exceeding the resources of the person.

Causalgia is a syndrome of sustained burning pain, allodynia, and hyperpathia after a traumatic nerve lesion, often combined with vasomotor and sudomotor dysfunction and later trophic changes.

Dysaesthesia is an unpleasant abnormal sensation, whether spontaneous or evoked.

Hyperalgesia is an increased response to a stimulus which is normally painful.

Hyperaesthesia is increased sensitivity to stimulation, excluding the special senses.

Individuate first described by Carl Gustav Jung as the process of becoming aware of oneself, of one's make-up, and the way to discover one's true, inner self.

Neuritis is inflammation of a nerve or nerves. (Note: Not to be used unless inflammation is thought to be present.)

Neurogenic pain is pain initiated or caused by a primary lesion, dysfunction, or transitory perturbation in the peripheral or central nervous system.

Neuropathic pain is pain initiated or caused by a primary lesion or dysfunction in the nervous system.

Nociceptor is a receptor preferentially sensitive to a noxious stimulus or to a stimulus which would become noxious if prolonged. When an injury occurs involving the nociceptors, nociceptive pain results, often described as aching or throbbing.

Noxious stimulus is one which is damaging to normal tissues. (Note: Although the definition of a noxious stimulus has been retained, the term is not used in this list to define other terms.)

Pain threshold is the least experience of pain which a subject can recognise.

Pain tolerance level is the greatest level of pain which a subject is prepared to tolerate.

Paraesthesia is an abnormal sensation, whether spontaneous or evoked.

Peripheral neurogenic pain is pain initiated or caused by a primary lesion or dysfunction or transitory perturbation in the peripheral nervous system.

Peripheral neuropathic pain is pain initiated or caused by a primary lesion or dysfunction in the peripheral nervous system.

Self-efficacy Perceived self-efficacy is concerned with people's judgement of their capabilities to execute given levels of performance and to exercise control over events. Judgements of self-efficacy affect what courses of action people choose to pursue; how much effort they will put forth in a given endeavour; how long they will persevere in the face of aversive experiences; whether their thought patterns help or hinder their endeavour; and how much stress they experience in coping with taxing environmental demands (Bandura, 1986).

Somataform pain disorder, a diagnostic category in DSM 1V in which there is a focus on pain, psychological component is felt to be primary and the organic involvement is either absent or minimal. *The Diagnostic and Statistical Manual of Mental Disorders* (DSM; American Psychiatric Association; 1994) describes somatisation disorder criteria being met before the age of 25 years, but symptoms often presenting in adolescence.

Values are 'chosen qualities of purposive action, which can only be instantiated rather than processed as an object' (Hayes and Strosahl, 2004).

References

Bandura A. *Social Foundations of Thought and Action: a social cognitive theory.* Englewood Cliffs, NJ: Prentice-Hall; 1986.

Diagnostic and Statistical Manual of Mental Disorders: DSM IV, 4th ed. Washington D.C: American Psychiatric Association; 1994.

Hayes SC, Strosahl KD, editors. *A Practical Guide to Acceptance and Commitment Therapy.* New York: Springer; 2004.

Lazarus RS, Folkman S. *Stress, Appraisal and Coping.* New York: Springer; 1984.

Taylor S. Anxiety sensitivity: theoretical perspectives and recent findings. *Behav Res Ther.* 1995: **33**: 243–58.

Appendix: The handouts

See www.radcliffe-oxford.com/adolescentpain

1 Strategies for sleep

These strategies have been found to be very useful in assisting people to sleep. They can be particularly helpful if you are experiencing pain which interferes with your sleep.

Preparing for sleep

☆ **Establish a routine.** If you go to bed at the same time every night, you are training your body to know when it should be ready to sleep. No matter how much sleep you have had, try to get up at the same time in the morning. Use an alarm clock for this. The body needs to experience hours of daylight in order to distinguish night from day, which triggers the message for sleep.

☆ **Keep to the routine even on weekends and holidays** if you are training yourself to establish a routine; you need to at least for a few months until your sleep habits are established. Staying up until after midnight will trigger the old learned habits of sleep difficulty. You may be able to sleep in, once you have retrained your body into the new habits for a sufficient period of time.

☆ **Sleeping in the daytime is not a good idea** as this confuses your body clock, and makes it more difficult to sleep at night.

☆ **Do some physical exercise during the day** (walking is especially good). This means you are physically, not just mentally, tired at the end of the day.

☆ **Avoid stimulants in the evenings**, e.g. drinking caffeine or alcohol. These inhibit getting to sleep. Instead, a small warm milk drink or herbal tea can help you to settle to sleep. You may have a light snack.

☆ **Keep your bed as a place for sleep, not anything else.** When you get into bed, say to yourself, 'Now I am going to sleep.' It is not a good idea to watch TV, talk on the phone, or do homework in bed. If you keep your bed for sleeping only, your body gets the message that when you get into bed it is time for sleep.

☆ **If you are unable to sleep after 10–15 minutes, get out of bed**, go to another room and do a quiet activity until you feel sleepy, then begin again. You may need to do this several times to start with.

☆ **Avoid stimulating activities near bedtime** such as exercise, having stimulating chats or arguments, eating heavy meals (a light snack is OK), or doing demanding intellectual work. Give yourself wind-down time. Calming activities that can help some people settle to sleep include: reading a book or magazine, listening to easy music or the radio, having a warm (not too hot) bath or shower. Try to notice any signs of tiredness in your body, as this is the best time to go to bed.

☆ **Use the relaxation strategies** you have learnt before you get into bed, or if you wake up during the night. Focus your mind and use breathing or mindfulness techniques to let go of any worries. Although this focus may seem difficult to start at night, it can be surprisingly more effective, especially if you have been practising at other times. If focus seems especially hard, limit yourself to 10 or 20 breaths to start. Mark these off by moving a finger with each breath. Don't use numbers to count, as this is distracting from the focus on breath. This is helpful in the middle of the night to assist getting back to sleep.

☆ **Use your imagination positively.** This is like creating your own movie (or dream) behind your eyes. Imagine a quiet place or activity you love, fill in all the physical details including colour, texture and smell of the place. Put yourself in this movie and freely move about. The place or activity you create can be whatever or wherever you want, in the country, by the sea, at home – what matters is that it is peaceful and feels safe and interesting to you.

☆ **Keep a notebook by the bed**, so if your thoughts are racing or worrying, you can write them down. Tell yourself that it is unlikely that you will find a solution right now and that your mind is just on repetitive 'tram tracks'. It's OK to stop thinking about them now because you can think about them in the morning when you are more likely to find a solution.

Remember

☆ If you don't sleep tell yourself it is OK. Whilst lying in bed your body is resting and you will be all right in the morning.

☆ Make sure clock faces are not visible so that you are not 'clock watching'.

☆ A routine may take several months of persistent practice to establish.

☆ In general, no harm will occur if you do not sleep for one or two nights. Remember you are still resting and you will catch up on sleep later because you are tired.

☆ Accept that progress may be slow, especially if the problem has been there a while. If it seems hard and you are losing heart, keep a log of your sleeping patterns and compare them with your earlier baseline. You can gradually move your going-to-bed time back by 15 minutes at a time for a week or so. To keep yourself on track, record whatever factors are affecting your sleep, such as difficulty getting to sleep, how long you slept for, how many times you woke in the night, and how you felt when waking up in the morning.

☆ If sleep issues or pain are extreme or continue to get worse, you may benefit from visiting a sleep clinic or discussing with your pain specialist doctor pain medications that can also assist sleep. But remember that medications are only a short-term answer; retraining yourself is the long-term solution.

2   Imagining a special place

This is like being the director of your own movie. You decide the scene and the action. You will need to include lots of details to make it come alive. Remember your movie is for the purpose of relaxation and distraction for you, so choose a place and activity that you love and feel safe in. You can do this in a chair or lying down.

☆ Choose a special place (or activity).
☆ Ideas: backyard, beach, waterfall, forest, cooking, walking, your grandmother's house, etc.
☆ Make yourself comfortable so that you can be still. Close your eyes.
☆ Begin to **imagine**. Start to **notice** details: what is in your picture (e.g. trees, flowers, ground etc)? Are there colours, what is above you? Notice the smells, sounds, and textures.
☆ Begin to **imagine** yourself moving through this special place. What do you encounter?
☆ **Explore** this special place and anything that happens in it.
☆ This is the beginning of entering your private dream world.

If you are lying down you may fall asleep. If not, to come away from your special place, give yourself a few moments to tune into where you are. Do this by starting to hear the sounds around you and picturing the room or place where you are at this moment.

3 Do's and don'ts for . . . . .'s family!

The 'do's and don'ts' below have been discussed with . . . . . . and she/he understands why they are useful for him/her. You don't have to believe in them immediately just to keep doing them. As . . . . . . learns to manage herself/himself, everyone will feel more confident. Everyone may take some time to feel comfortable and successful with these new ways of being together and remember, you don't have to be perfect! (If can be helpful to discuss your feelings of discomfort with your therapist.)

☆ Believe that . . . . . . has real pain but that you are not responsible for relieving it.

☆ It is not helpful to ask her/him about her pain. Comforting her/him takes away her sense of her own ability, she has thought about this but may take some time to believe it 100%!

☆ Don't offer help especially to get things for her/him . . . . . . is learning to be independent in her/his management.

☆ If she/he asks for help it is OK to say to her/him 'Is that something you can take charge of yourself?' . . . . . . knows that this is her/his cue to consider what she/he can do for herself.

☆ . . . . . . is not going to use resting with Mum, or with others, as a way of managing pain or having an enjoyable time. She/he has chosen to have activity as fun, e.g. cooking or shopping.

☆ A heat pack and rest is not a pain-management tool.

☆ Life-engaging activity, including school attendance, is a distraction and a pain-management tool.

☆ If . . . . . . is at a loss as to what to do, he/she can refer to his book from the therapy sessions.

☆ . . . . . . may reward herself/himself for her/his independent pain-management activity by having a heat pack, e.g. after having done the relaxation or mindfulness, the diary record, etc.

☆ . . . . . . can add to this list if she/he feels there may be some things that will be helpful for her/his independence.

4   Managing pain behaviours

Pain behaviour is associated with increasing the areas in the brain that are responsive to pain, thereby increasing sensitivity to pain. In other words, decreasing pain behaviour decreases the experience of pain.

Positive reinforcement is a response to your child's behaviour that will increase the likelihood of the behaviour occurring again. **Attention** for pain behaviour is a very powerful reinforcer for children.

☆ Emphasise that you are unable to take your child's pain away, but say that she/he will receive lots of love and attention (not about pain or pain behaviour) and given rewards for coping.

☆ Ignore any pain behaviours exhibited by your child (verbal groaning, crying, guarding).

☆ Give special attention and praise for coping behaviours (relaxation and breathing techniques have been taught, along with visualisation).

☆ Do not enter into a discussion with your child regarding her pain and function, e.g. walk away.

Do . . .

☆ give attention during symptom-free periods (e.g. 'you are working well', and 'you are doing well')

☆ be aware of demands for positioning; they are probably requests for attention

☆ expect your child to function in spite of physical distress (this is not cruel but actually therapeutic as your child will be convinced of their ability to manage by the experience of success)

☆ be firm – this communicates the conviction that your child is strong enough and competent enough to overcome this distress

☆ believe that your child can increase her functioning

☆ treat your child as an active agent in her treatment

☆ help your child to problem solve about how to actively change things, e.g. 'what can you do about this?'

☆ reduce parental concern if the opportunity arises

☆ be aware of how you feel towards your child

☆ follow through with times and expectations put into place

☆ support all members of the treating team.

Do not . . .

☆ assume responsibility for anything your child can do themself
☆ use punishment or assess their progress negatively in front of your child
☆ focus on the illness behaviours or give attention for pain behaviour
☆ ask how she/he is feeling or how much pain she/he has
☆ give excessive reassurance
☆ focus attention on the symptoms or show concern (even though you may feel it!)
☆ attend to your child when she/he is in pain or in discomfort
☆ believe your child is vulnerable and unable to cope.

(*Courtesy of Sophia Franks*)

5 Using breath to find ease in movement

We unconsciously 'read' our body sensations and interpret with thoughts, i.e. if our heart races and we feel this as fear, our unconscious thoughts are likely to also match this interpretation, 'something dangerous is happening'. A similar fear response is possible with our breath. Remember what happens when you get a fright – a sharp intake of air that is held ('I didn't dare to breathe!'). Sometimes when pain occurs, it seems natural to avoid it by holding your breath to endure it by 'grinning and bearing it' and not looking or feeling where it is. However if the pain doesn't lessen, this can contribute to a sense of fear and avoidance of the place of hurt. Knowing how to **breathe with ease around the pain, avoids the association of increasing fear that can come in avoiding the area**. It's a little bit like looking a bully in the face and saying 'I'm not afraid of you!'

This looking-the-pain-bully in the face, is not the same as focusing on the pain (you are usually recommended not to focus on pain). This strategy arms you with techniques that give positive feelings and images that focus on **enjoyment rather than fear** of the body.

When you breathe in you contract and shorten the breathing muscles – when you breathe out you release the contraction, relax the muscles which lengthen and soften. **When you breathe out you are actually relaxing the diaphragm**, the largest breathing muscle in the middle of your body. Learning to **'let go'** effort and tension in breathing makes it easy to transfer this feeling to other parts of the body. Learning to use this as a conscious process means you can **'turn on' ease** in your body when you need it. Being relaxed also releases endorphins, your body's natural painkillers.

First practise easy breath

☆ You can feel your diaphragm best when lying on the floor on your back. Place your hand on your tummy just below your ribs and above your navel. Feel how your hand lifts up when you breathe in. That's your diaphragm pressing down, causing your hand to lift up.

☆ Take time to practise focusing on this during the day, at times when you are not exercising or moving. At this time, focus on the sensation of the out-breath, the heaviness, stillness, etc. **Train yourself by saying as you breathe out – 'relax'**. . . feel the shoulders drop . . . etc., until the feeling of relaxing becomes familiar. You can feel this best at the **very end** of the out-breath just before the new in-breath, when there is a still moment when all the air is gone. Notice this moment when you are most relaxed: even the breathing muscles are still. The middle of the body needs to feel soft so don't use force by pushing or holding air out.

Breathing and moving with ease

Practitioners of yoga learn to use breath as part of their practice. These principles are based on that practice and can be applied to any movements.

☆ When exercising or moving, use the 'letting go' feeling of relaxation on the out-breath that you have learned, to relax at **the end of a muscle contraction**. That is, breathe out when you return to easy position, e.g. when your arms return to rest at the side of your body or you return your legs to the resting position. Remember the empty end of the breath is the best moment to savour relaxing. Take time to plan the breathing that is best for each exercise. Practise working out when is the right moment to breath in, and when to breathe out, and learn to establish the ease and a comfortable rhythm.

☆ Usually the **in-breath goes with the muscle effort and the out-breath when you release the effort**. If you are in a held position, e.g. a stretch, you can use the out-breath to make it easier.

☆ Consciously **send your in-breath down lower in the body, engaging the diaphragm** and feeling the pushing down into the abdomen. Never hold air in, in the upper chest.

☆ If you **experience pain in a stretch you can use this deeper breathing** to emphasise the relaxing, letting-go of the out-breath to release where it is tight – breath into the tight area, say to yourself *'expand, let go'*. Start with just a few out-breaths during the stretch increasing them gradually as you acquire ease.

☆ **Use your imagination to picture the place where the stretch or discomfort exists.** Imagine fibres of a tight rope loosening and creating space between each fibre with each out-breath. You are creating space.

☆ It is best not to **expect** the breath to send the pain away, as this leads to feelings of failure. This may or may not happen, simply accept what is there. Breath may change the pain but more importantly, it will allow you to feel good about your management and easier in your body, and it will allow you to increase your range of movement and function.

6   Easy breathing practice

☆ Start lying flat out on the floor with flat hands on your tummy. Notice that when you breathe in, your tummy rises up and lifts your hands.

☆ Every time you notice your hands rise up on the in-breath, move one finger sideways. This is a way of noting each breath without having to count. Move one finger sideways for each breath until all fingers are moved (this will be 10 breaths). Do this again if you feel OK.

☆ Then focus your mind particularly on breathing out, noticing that there is a space at the end of the out-breath.

☆ With eyes closed, see if you can watch this empty space, when there is no breath. Just for a moment, you feel soft in the tummy, heavy and still all over. Say to yourself, 'Let go, relax.' Breath in when you need to again.

☆ Never hold the air out so that it is difficult or a struggle. If this happens, stop doing it.

☆ After this time, focus on feeling heavy in each arm then in the legs, then the hips, shoulders, head, etc.

☆ At the end, feel your whole body completely relaxed in one piece. Allow yourself to open your eyes slowly and to feel how your body has changed. Take your time and move slowly to keep the feeling. **Notice what has changed since you began.**

7 Owning helpful thoughts

You are probably aware of which unhelpful self-talk you experience. Look through the following and identify for yourself which ones will help you to take charge and turn these negative unhelpful thoughts into helpful ones that will help you move forward.

☆ When I do my exercises I am taking control.
☆ Instead of asking 'why', it's there, I can take action to manage it.
☆ I am in charge of my health.
☆ Relaxation is a natural pain killer.
☆ I can choose to stop before overdoing it.
☆ My pain is not damage.
☆ Pain flare-ups come but they also go away.
☆ Pain can be unpredictable but I can manage it whenever it comes.
☆ If I keep moving I will keep myself fit.
☆ Resting is not the best pain-management strategy.
☆ I can manage pain by persisting with tasks and using relaxation/ breathing.
☆ I can choose the direction of my life.
☆ Pain is inevitable but not invincible.
☆ I don't have to be perfect.
☆ I can talk myself through fear.
☆ Getting angry just makes the pain worse.
☆ I can breathe into my anger.
☆ When I am worried I can ask for help.
☆ Nobody else can take my pain away.
☆ I am the only person who can take action when pain happens.

8 Learning to focus

Don't start with expectations of how good or bad you might be. Relaxation/mindfulness or task persistence doesn't happen by magic, it's a process and a skill to be learned like any other.

Start with achievable, small steps, e.g. if focusing on breath, limit it to five breaths that you mark up by moving a finger for each breath. Add five more as you feel more confident. You may want to start these at first with your eyes open then try five or so with your eyes closed.

Be like a mother who is kind to a wandering toddler. Be gentle but insist that you guide it in the direction you want to go. Simply notice what distracted you and go back to the details of your task. If you get cross, the toddler has won! Persevere and notice your achievements after every session.

The best way to help a wandering mind is to occupy it. One way is to be **very, very** interested in the details of what you are doing. In breathing, think about what it feels like inside your body at the moment of each breath, what sensations are there. Focus on each breath as if it is the first breath you have ever taken. When doing a task, notice the details of what you are doing, the colour, smell, textures, movements required, etc. Focus on it as if you have to describe the experience to another person.

9 Diaphragm breathing exercise

a Lying on the floor

Remove your shoes. Loosen any tight-fitting items of clothing from around your neck or waist. Lie on your back on a firm surface (not *in* bed). You may find it more comfortable to complete the exercise in a warm room or with a blanket as your body temperature lowers when you are lying still. You may like to support your head with a pillow. It is best to lie symmetrically, with your legs out and feet slightly apart. Alternatively, you may prefer to have your knees bent with feet about hip-width apart. A pillow can be used to prop up the legs.

Close your eyes and bring your attention to your breathing. Notice the sensation of breathing in and out. Feel the air passing through the nostrils. Notice it is cool on the in-breath and warm on the out-breath. Be interested in every detail and sensation.

If you find your mind wanders, notice that it has and gently bring it back to the task. No matter how many times you need to do this, do it without judging yourself.

Place both your hands gently on your abdomen. Inhale slowly and deeply through your nose into your abdomen to push up your hands as much as feels comfortable. Your chest should only move a little. If this exercise becomes uncomfortable or makes you feel tense, just focus on your normal breathing pattern. You might like to place one hand on your chest and one hand on your abdomen and just feel your hands rise and fall (with the little finger on top of your navel).

Continue to take in long, deep, slow breaths. Focus on the feeling of breathing out; notice the feeling of softening in the abdomen as you breath out; let the sinking, softening feeling there last for as long as is comfortable. You may notice a special moment when there is no air, and that you are quite still. At this special moment even your breathing muscles are relaxed. You are at your most relaxed. Stay with that moment, watch it, allow it to stay for as long as is comfortable, i.e. until you naturally breathe in. Do not hold the air out as this will become uncomfortable. Your relaxing out-breath will gradually lengthen in this process.

Notice the changed sensation within your body when you are relaxed. Continue for as long as you like. At the end of the exercise, spend a little time appreciating the sensation of relaxation so that you can take it with you!

b In a chair or walking

You can do modified versions of the above script for sitting in a chair, or even for walking. In these positions, the experience is different so it is important not to expect the same outcome. Because the seated position squashes the abdominal area, it is more difficult to feel the diaphragm moving the lower abdomen. It is easier to feel the shoulders and ribs sinking as you breathe out, so this sensation is also a useful area for focus. If concentration is difficult, you may like to restrict your practice to just ten breaths by moving one finger for each breath. In this way you are still able to focus on the sensations of relaxing rather than trying to remember to count.

10 Mindfulness meditation

It is important to practise mindfulness in everyday activities as well as at times when unpleasant internal events occur.

Noticing five things

This is a simple exercise to centre yourself, and connect with your environment. Practise it throughout the day, especially at any time you find yourself getting caught up in your thoughts and feelings.

☆ Pause for a moment.
☆ Notice five things you can see.
☆ Notice five things you can hear.
☆ Notice five things you can feel in contact with your body (e.g. your feet in your shoes, the air on your face, your back against the chair and the fabric of your clothes touching your legs).

This is a good exercise to use when walking to school or even in class.

Mindfulness of a task

Pick an activity you do every day. It may be cleaning your teeth, making your bed, washing the dishes. Notice every detail involved in this task. If you are cleaning your teeth, notice exactly what your toothbrush looks like as you place the toothpaste on it; its colour, the shape of the bristles, the spaces between them, then the shape and colour of the paste and the smell that comes with it. When you put it in your mouth notice the sensations that occur, the taste, temperature, saliva, your tongue, etc. If you get bored or frustrated, simply notice what you're feeling and bring your attention back to the task and the details you can notice.

Again and again, your mind will wander. As soon as you notice this, gently notice what distracted you and bring your attention back to your current activity.

This is useful to do in class if pain interrupts your concentration.

Observe, breathe, expand, allow

This exercise employs some of the breath awareness and detachment or defusion exercises described earlier. It is important to understand at the beginning that these exercises are not intended to control, remove or diminish your negative private events although they may change over time. You can use this exercise to gradually increase your tolerance to, and acceptance of unpleasant sensations or thoughts while still persisting with your chosen tasks.

While you are pursuing values or goal-based activity, you may experience any unpleasant private event (e.g. an increase in pain, or anxiety). If this would normally cause you to withdraw from the activity you may try the following:

☆ Observe the details of the sensation or thought. Notice where it is in the body; does it move, throb; does it have a definition, shape, colour or texture; write the words up on a screen?

☆ Breathe into the area around the sensation or words and into the shape itself.

☆ Expand: make space around it to make room for it.

☆ Accept that it is there and allow it to be there, saying 'I don't like this feeling but I have room for it' or 'It's unpleasant but I can accept it' or 'Just notice it and move on.'

A useful acronym to remember the process is OBEA. (O is for observe, B is for breathe, E is for expand, A is for accept.)

11 Record of practice

Instructions

This record is primarily for your benefit so you can keep track of when you have practised. Record when you have done practice at the end of each day. It can be helpful to note the time. Initially, learning relaxation/mindfulness requires a short burst of intense learning, so aim for at least three practices of any length. Regularity and frequency of practice are more important than the length of each one. If you start with one and your record shows you are gradually managing to add one more, you are on the right track. The more you do it, the better you will be at it. Build it into your daily routine and activities, for example in class, as a passenger in the bus or car or on the way to school. In particular, practise it when you notice a familiar trigger for an unpleasant sensation, thought or feeling – including when, because of pain, you want to avoid an activity that you are fit enough to do.

☆ Fill in days of the week.

☆ Place a tick (or the time of day) for each relaxation/mindfulness session.

☆ Record events that triggered unpleasant sensations (e.g. pain), thoughts or feelings where you used the technique in the challenges column.

☆ Full regular practice is best.

☆ Remember, relaxation takes practice, the more regularly you do it, the easier it becomes.

Record of practice

Start date: _____   *Name:* _____

DAY	UP TO 20 MINS	UP TO 5 MINS	UP TO 5 MINS	UP TO 5 MINS	UP TO 5 MINS	CHALLENGES/TRIGGERS
1						
2						
3						
4						
5						
6						
7						
8						
9						
10						
11						
12						
13						
14						

12 Examples of a thought diary

Example 1

INCIDENT OR ACTIVITY	BODILY REACTION	EMOTIONS OR FEELINGS	THOUGHTS	ACTION	ALTERNATIVE ACTION	ALTERNATIVE THOUGHT; % BELIEF

Example 2

EVENT	BODY SENSATIONS	EMOTIONS	THOUGHT	ACTION CONTEMPLATED	BEHAVIOUR	CONSEQUENCES	ALTERNATIVE ACTION	ALTERNATIVE CONSEQUENCES

Index